Culinary dictionary for corticosteroid therapy

MENARD Cédric
DIETICIAN-NUTRITIONIST

© 2020, Cédric MENARD

All rights reserved

ISBN: 9798697186527

Traduced by Mélanie GEFFROY

Corticosteroid therapy

Nutrition is as **fundamentally** important if your doctor uses corticosteroid therapy to treat your pathology. You then have to greatly decrease your sodium and sugar intakes and increase your calcium, vitamin D and protein intakes.

Note: this book is suitable for oral corticotherapy exclusively in the case of rheumatic, respiratory, or immune diseases, as well as in the case of eye diseases. However, this book is not suitable for inflammatory colitis, as well as for most cancers treated with corticotherapy.

Legend of this book

- The searched word is **consumable** or applicable (if it's a culinary technique) <u>**without any restriction, insofar as it has not undergone any change from its initial state before consumption**</u>, and even plays a positive role in the context of your corticotherapy. In this case, it will be accompanied by **four full stars ★★★★**.

- The searched word is **consumable** or applicable (if it's a culinary technique) <u>**without any restriction**</u> because of its low or lack of sodium and sugar contributions, <u>**insofar as it has not undergone any modification of its initial state before its consumption**</u>, but its role remains neutral. In this case, it will be accompanied by **three full stars ★★★**.

- The searched word is **consumable** or applicable (if it's a culinary technique) <u>**only under certain conditions, in particular if the food is neither salty nor sweet**</u>, which will be annotated. In this case, it will be accompanied by **two stars full ★★**.

- The searched word is **edible, but in great moderation**. In this case, it will have **one full star★**. In the best case scenario, do not eat it.

> - The searched word is **greatly not recommended**, not to say forbidden. It will be designated by this type of grey frame.

Note: many of the foods known as "Low sodium", "Salt-free", "No salt", "Low in salt", **and/or**, "Sugar-free", etc. are not listed in this book. Obviously, they are, by definition, perfectly consumable as part of your diet under corticotherapy, **if and only if they are both sugar-free <u>and</u> salt-free!**

7

A

Abalone/*Ormeau*: edible saltwater mollusk.

Abondance cheese /*Abondance*: semi-hard and raw cow's milk cheese.

Accra★★/*Acra*: croquette of crushed cod or other various elements coated with fritter batter and fried in boiling oil.
Note: many commercially prepared foods are high in salt: prepare it yourself without salt and with authorized foods.

Achars★★/*Achards*: Indian condiment made of fruits and vegetables macerated in vinegar.
Note: many commercially prepared foods are high in salt: prepare it yourself without salt and with authorized foods.

Adzuki bean/*Haricot azukis*: cf. "Kidney bean".

Adzuki flake★★★/*Flocon d'azukis*: small portion of dehydrated adzuki. Gluten-free.

Agar-agar★★★/*Agar-agar*: mucilage made from seaweed used as setting agent.

Agave syrup/*Sirop d'agave*: syrup considered as a sweetener made of agave.

Aiguillette★★/*Aiguillette*: beef meat to roast. Red meat.

Aillade/*Aillade*: bread crouton rubbed with garlic and moistened with olive oil. Carbohydrate.

Alcohol (alcoholic beverage)★/*Alcool (boisson alcoolisée)*: wine, liqueur, beer, etc. made from alcohol fermentation.
Note: do not drink alcoholic beverage, however no problem if it's cooked.

9

Alcohol-free beer★/*Bière sans alcool*: drink from the alcoholic fermentation of mainly barley and from which the alcohol is extracted.

Alexanders★★★/*Maceron*: plant from which we eat the young blanched shoots. Green vegetable.

Alfalfa seed★★★/*Graine d'alfalfa*: alfalfa seeds eaten crushed or germinated.

Alliaria★★★/*Alliaire*: plant with white flowers, garlic scent and spicy taste.

Almond★★★/*Amande*: seed of the almond tree.

Almond butter★★★/*Beurre d'amande*: food paste made of grilled almonds.

Almond cream★★★/*Crème d'amande*: more or less liquid cream made of almond milk, substitute to crème fraîche.

Almond milk★★/*Lait d'amande*: plant milk from almonds. Lactose-free.
Note: do not consume it sweetened.

Almond milk cream dessert/*Crème dessert au lait d'amande*: vegetable dessert made of almond milk, sugar and eggs. Dairy product.

Almond milk yogurt/*Yaourt au lait d'amande*: almond milk fermented thanks to lactic acid bacteria, sweetened or not. Dairy product. Lactose-free.

Almond oil★★★/*Huile d'amande*: fatty substance made of almond.

Almond pasta★★★/*Pâte alimentaire à base d'amande*: mix to be cooked made of sieved almond flour. Gluten-free.

Almond purée★★★/***Purée d'amande***: mashed almonds to spread.

Almond seed★★★/***Graine d'amande***: almond seed eaten crushed or germinated.

Almond syrup★★/***Orgeat***: almond milk with orange blossom.
Note: do not consume it sweetened.

Amandine/*Amandine*: almond tartlet.

Amaranth★★★/***Amarante***: vegetable plant from which we eat the young leaves. Green vegetable.

Amaranth flour★★★/***Farine d'amarante***: powder made of not wholewheat amaranth milling. Gluten-free.

Amaranth pasta★★★/***Pâte alimentaire à base d'amarante***: mix to be cooked made of not whole-grain amaranth flour. Gluten-free.

Amaranth seed★★★/***Graine d'amarante***: amaranth seed eaten crushed or germinated.

American cheese: melted cheese. Dairy product.

Anchoïade★★/***Anchoïade***: anchovy and olive oil purée.
Note: many commercially prepared foods are high in salt: prepare it yourself without salt and with authorized foods.

Anchovy★★/**Anchois**: small fatty saltwater fish.
Note: only if it's unsalted.

Anchovy cream★★/***Crème d'anchois***: mixed anchovies with olive oil.
Note: many commercially prepared foods are high in salt: prepare it yourself without salt and with authorized foods.

Anchovy in oil★★/*Anchois à l'huile***: anchovy fillet preserved in vegetable oil.
Note: only if it's unsalted.

Andouille/*Andouille***: product made of cooked cold meat, wrapped in black entrails, especially made from pork.

Andouillette/*Andouillette***: cooked cold meat wrapped in entrails, especially made from pork.

Angelica★★★/*Angélique***: aromatic umbellifer plant.

Angler fish★★★/*Lotte***: saltwater or freshwater fish with white flesh.

Angler fish liver★★/*Foie de lotte***: liver of the angler fish, saltwater fish. Offal.
Note: only if it's unsalted.

Anise★★★/*Anis***: fruit used to flavor some alcoholic beverages, dishes, etc.

Appelwood cheese: raw or pasteurised cow's milk cheese. Dairy product.

Appenzeller cheese/*Appenzel***: hard cow's milk Swiss cheese. Dairy product.

Appetizer/*Amuse-gueule***: small salty cake, canapé, etc.

Apple in light syrup★/*Pomme au sirop léger***: poached apple preserved in more or less sugary water.

Apple in syrup/*Pomme au sirop***: poached apple preserved in very sugary water.

Apple juice/*Jus de pomme***: juice made of the pressing of apples.

Apricot in light syrup★/*Abricot au sirop léger***: poached apricot preserved in more or less sugary water.

Apricot in syrup/*Abricot au sirop*: poached apricot preserved in very sugary water.

Apricot jelly/*Pâte d'abricot*: cf. "Dried apricot".

Apricot juice/Jus d'abricot: juice made of the pressing of apricots.

Arctic char★★★/*Omble*: fatty freshwater fish.

Arctostaphylos uva-ursi★★★/*Busserole*: small edible berry from a bush: the arctostaphylos uva-ursi tree. Fresh fruit.

Argan oil★★★/*Huile d'argan*: fatty substance made of argan.

Aronia in might syrup★/*Aronia au sirop léger*: poached aronia preserved in more or less sugary water.

Aronia in syrup/*Aronia au sirop*: poached aronia preserved in very sugary water.

Artichoke★★★/*Artichaut*: vegetable perennial plant grown for its flower heads from which we eat the bract. Green vegetable.
Note: do not eat canned vegetables (unless low in salt).

Arugula★★★/*Roquette*: annual plant from which the prickly leaves are eaten in salad. Green vegetable.

Arugula seed★★★/*Graine de roquette*: arugula seed eaten crushed or germinated.

Asiago/*Asiago*: Italian hard cow's milk cheese. Dairy product.

Asparagus★★★/*Asperge*: vegetable plant grown for its young shoots. Green vegetables.
Note: do not eat canned vegetables (unless low in salt).

Asparagus pea★★★/*Pois-asperge*: vegetable plant from which we eat the cloves and the seeds. Green vegetable.
Note: do not eat canned vegetables (unless low in salt).

Aspartame★★★/*Aspartame*: intense artificial sweetener with no calorie.

Aspic/*Aspic*: dish coated with jelly.

Asses' milk★★★/*Lait d'ânesse*: whole milk from the she-ass.

Atlantic horse mackerel★★★/*Chinchard*: fatty saltwater fish.

Atriplex hortensis★★★/*Arroche*: plant with triangular leaves. Only one species is edible. Green vegetable.

Avocado★★★/*Avocat*: oleaginous fruit of the avocado tree.

Avocado oil★★★/*Huile d'avocat*: fatty substance made of avocado.

Ayrshire cheese: raw or pasteurised cow's milk cheese. Dairy product.

Azerole in light syrup★/*Azerole au sirop léger*: poached azerole preserved in more or less sugary water.

Azerole in powder★★★/*Azerole en poudre*: azerole extracts sold in capsules or in tablets.

Azerole in syrup/*Azerole au sirop*: poached azerole preserved in sugary water.

ℬ

Babelutte/*Babelutte*: candy cane flavored with honey or brown sugar.

Baby-beef★★/*Baby-beef*: young bovine fattened for its meat, slaughtered between 12 and 15 months. Red meat.

Bacon/*Bacon*: piece of pork carcass salted and smoked, cut in thin slices. Cooked meat.

Bagel/*Bagel*: small white bread shaped into a ring with very firm crumb. Carbohydrate.

Bagnes cheese/*Bagnes*: hard unpasteurized cow's milk cheese. Dairy product.

Baguette/*Baguette*: white bread that has a high glycemic index. Carbohydrate.

Baker's yeast★★★/*Levure de boulanger*: unicellular microscopic mushrooms used for the bread batter fermentation.

Baking powder/*Levure chimique*: mix of chemical products used in pastry cooking and in cookie cooking to make the batter rise.

Baking soda/*Bicarbonate de soude*: cf. "Bicarbonate of soda".

Baklava/*Baklava*: small Turkish cake with puff pastry, honey and almonds.

Ballan wrasse★★★/*Vieille*: saltwater fish with white flesh.

Ballotine/*Ballottine*: rolled galantine with poultry and stuffing. Cooked meat.

Bambara nut★★★/*Pois de bambara*: ground-bean. Carbohydrate. Gluten-free.
Note: do not eat canned vegetables (unless low in salt).

Bamboo (shoot of)★★★/*Bambou (pousses de)*: young shoots of edible bamboo. Green vegetable.
Note: do not eat canned vegetables (unless low in salt).

Banana juice/*Jus de banane*: juice made of the pressing of bananas. Exotic fruit.

Banana split/*Banana split*: dessert made of banana, vanilla ice cream, whipped cream and almonds. Exotic fruit.

Banana★★/*Banane tigrée*: tropical fruit of the banana tree, rich in starch before its full ripeness. Exotic fruit.
Note: consume it immediately after the meal.

Banon cheese/*Banon*: unpasteurized goat or sheep milk wrapped in a sweet chestnut leaf. Dairy product.

Barb★★★/*Barbeau*: freshwater fish with white flesh.

Barbecue sauce/*Sauce barbecue*: sauce mainly made of sugar, flavors and tomato purée.

Bard★★★/*Barde*: lard slice used to wrap a piece of poultry or a piece of meat.

Barley flake★★★/*Flocon d'orge*: small portion of dehydrated barley. Carbohydrate.

Barley milk★★/*Lait d'orge*: plant milk from barley. Lactose-free.
Note: do not consume it sweetened.

Barley milk cream dessert/*Crème dessert au lait d'orge*: vegetable dessert made of barley milk, sugar and eggs. Dairy product.

Barley pasta★★★/*Pâte alimentaire d'orge*: mix to be cooked made of refined barley flour. Carbohydrate.

Barracuda★★★/*Barracuda*: saltwater fish with white flesh.

Basil★★★/*Basilic*: herb you can use as a condiment.

Basil seed★★★/*Graine de basilic*: basil seed eaten crushed or germinated.

Basquaise sauce★★/*Sauce basquaise*: sauce made of tomatoes, onions, bell peppers, olives and Espelette chili peppers.
Note: many commercially prepared foods are high in salt: prepare it yourself without salt and with authorized foods.

Bass★★/*Bar*: saltwater fish with white flesh.

Batavia lettuce★★★/*Batavia*: lettuce with crunchy leaves. Green vegetable.

Bavarian cream★★/*Bavarois*: dessert with custard and gelatin.
Note: many commercially prepared foods are high in salt: prepare it yourself without salt and sugar and with authorized foods.

Bay★★★/*Laurier-sauce*: aromatic leaf used as a condiment.

Bearnaise sauce★★/*Sauce béarnaise*: sauce made of egg yolks, garlics, shallots, tarragons and butter.
Note: many commercially prepared foods are high in salt: prepare it yourself without salt and with authorized foods.

Beaufort cheese/*Beaufort*: firm raw cow's milk cheese. Dairy product.

Béchamel sauce - Beef short ribs

Béchamel sauce★★/*Sauce béchamel*: white sauce made of a roux and milk.
Note: many commercially prepared foods are high in salt: prepare it yourself without salt and with authorized foods.

Beef breast★★/*Poitrine de bœuf*: inferior part of the beef's rib cage to boil. Red meat.

Beef carpaccio★★/*Carpaccio de bœuf*: beef meat cut in very thin slices eaten raw, with a drop of olive oil and lemon juice. Red meat.

Beef cheek★★/*Joue de bœuf*: tender piece of beef cooked in sauce. Red meat.

Beef fondue★★/*Fondue bourguignonne*: dish made of small dices of beef dipped in boiling oil. Red meat.

Beef gristle★★/*Tendron de bœuf*: part of the beef composed of the cartilages which prolong the ribs. Red meat.

Beef kidney/*Rognon de bœuf*: kidney of the beef. Offal.

Beef knuckle★★/*Jarret de bœuf*: part of the leg behind the beef's knee joint. Meat to boil. Red meat.

Beef liver★★/*Foie de bœuf*: offal.

Beef (meat)/*Bœuf (viande de)*: all unprepared nor transformed meats, plain, ready to be cooked and cut from beef. See each piece separately.

Beef ravioli/*Ravioli de bœuf*: small square of pasta stuffed with beef meat, ground herbs, etc. before being poached. Carbohydrate.

Beef short ribs★★/*Plat de côte (de bœuf)*: beef meat to boil.

18

Beef spare rib★★/*Echine de bœuf*: part of the beef consisting of the ribs and the sirloin. Red meat.

Beef spider steak★★/*Araignée de bœuf*: piece of very tender meat from the beef's pelvis muscles. Red meat.

Beef steak★★/*Bifteck*: slice of beef to grill. Red meat.

Beef stock★★/*Fond de bœuf*: brown stock made of beef stock.
Note: many commercially prepared foods are high in salt: prepare it yourself without salt and with authorized foods.

Beef surlonge★★/*Surlonge de bœuf*: piece of beef to simmer. Red meat.

Beef tongue/*Langue de bœuf*: beef tongue eaten boiled. Offal.

Beef tournedos★★/*Tournedos de bœuf*: round slice of beef fillet. Red meat.

Beer★/*Bière*: beverage from alcoholic fermentation, especially barley alcoholic fermentation.
Note: do not drink alcoholic beverage, however no problem if it's cooked.

Beet★★★/*Betterave*: vegetable plant from which we eat the plump root. Green vegetable.
Note: do not eat canned vegetables (unless low in salt).

Beetroot chips/*Chips de betterave*: very thinly cut beetroots, fried and salted.

Beet seed★★★/*Graine de betterave*: beet seed eaten crushed or germinated.

Bell pepper/*Poivron*: soft bell pepper. Green vegetable.

Bicarbonate of soda/*Bicarbonate de sodium*: basic sodium salt sometimes used to ease stomach aches.

Bison (meat)★★/*Bison (viande de)*: meat very similar to that of beef. Red meat.

Bisque/*Bisque*: soup made of crustacean coulis.

Black ascophyllum/*Goémon noir*: edible seaweed.

Blackberry in light syrup★/*Mûre au sirop léger*: poached blackberry preserved in more or less sugary water.

Blackberry in syrup/*Mûre au sirop*: poached blackberry preserved in very sugary water.

Black bread/*Pain noir*: bread made of wheat flour, buckwheat flour, rye flour. Carbohydrate.

Blackcurrant in light syrup★/*Cassis au sirop léger*: poached blackcurrant preserved in more or less sugary water.

Blackcurrant in syrup/*Cassis au sirop*: poached blackcurrant preserved in very sugary water.

Black radish seed★★★/*Graine de radis noir*: black radish seed eaten crushed or germinated.

Black sausage/*Boudin noir*: cooked cold meat made of pork blood and fat stuffed in an intestine.

Black tea★★★/*Thé noir*: infusion of tea bush leaves lightly fermented after being picked.
Note: do not drink it sweetened.

Black turtle bean★★★/*Haricot noir*: black bean seed eaten fully ripe. Carbohydrate.

Blanquette★★/*Blanquette*: dish made of boiled meat (veal, turkey, lamb) served with a sauce made of stock thickened with flour and butter.
Note: many commercially prepared foods are high in salt: prepare it yourself without salt and with authorized foods.

Bleak★★★/*Ablette*: small freshwater fish with white flesh.

Blended yogurt/*Yaourt brassé*: cf. "Yogurt".

Blengdale blue: raw or pasteurised cow's milk cheese. Dairy product.

Bleu de Gex/*Septmoncel*: cow's milk cheese with mildew in it.

Bleu du Vercors-Sassenage/*Sassenage*: hard cow's milk cheese with internal mildew. Dairy product.

Bliblis★★/*Bliblis*: grilled chickpeas. Carbohydrate. Gluten-free.
Note: many commercially prepared foods are high in salt: prepare it yourself without salt and with authorized foods.

Blinis★★/*Blini*: small wheat and buckwheat crepe. Carbohydrate.
Note: many commercially prepared foods are high in salt: prepare it yourself without salt and with authorized foods.

Blitum bonus-henricus★★★/*Ansérine bon-henri*: vegetable plant from which we eat the young leaves. Green vegetable.

Blonchester cheese: raw or pasteurised cow's milk cheese. Dairy product.

Blood orange/*Orange sanguine*: cf. "Orange".

Blood orange juice/*Jus d'orange sanguine*: juice made of the pressing of blood oranges.

Bloody Mary/*Bloody Mary*: cocktail with vodka and tomato juice.

Blueberry in light syrup★/*Myrtille au sirop léger*: poached blueberry preserved in more or less sugary water.

Blueberry in syrup/*Myrtille au sirop*: poached blueberry preserved in very sugary water.

Blueberry juice/*Jus de myrtille*: juice made of the pressing of blueberries.

Blue cheese/*Bleu*: blue-veined aged cheese. Dairy product. Blue marble Jack, Maytag blue...

Blue marble Jack: pasteurised cow's milk cheese. Dairy product.

Boeuf bourguignon★★/*Bourguignon (bœuf)*: beef stew with red wine and onions. Red meat.
Note: many commercially prepared foods are high in salt: prepare it yourself without salt and with authorized foods.

Bogue★★★/*Bogue*: saltwater fish with white flesh.

Bolognese sauce★★/*Sauce bolognaise*: sauce made of tomatoes, onions and ground meat (usually beef meat, so red meat).
Note: many commercially prepared foods are high in salt: prepare it yourself without salt and with authorized foods.

Borage★★★/*Bourrache officinale*: plant you can use as condiment and from which we eat the young leaves.

Bouillabaisse/*Bouillabaisse*: soup made of various fish, crustacea, etc.

Brains★★★/*Cervelle*: brain of some animals intended to be eaten.

Braised (cooking method)★★/*Braisé (cuisson en)*: cooking method consisting in cooking food in a very flavored and low-fat or even no fat at all base, in isolation.
Note: many commercially prepared foods are high in salt: prepare it yourself without salt and with authorized foods.

Braised ham/*Jambon braisé*: pork ham juged in a braising base.

Bran bread/*Pain de son*: cf. "Wholewheat bread".

Brandade★★/*Brandade*: dish made of cod and potatoes.
Note: many commercially prepared foods are high in salt: prepare it yourself without salt and with authorized foods.

Brazil nut/*Noix du Brésil*: cf. "Nut".

Bread★★/*Paner*: to coat a food with a mixture of whipped egg and breadcrumbs before cooking it.
Note: many commercially prepared foods are high in salt: prepare it yourself without salt and with authorized foods.

Breadcrumbs/*Chapelure*: white bread toasted in the oven before being crushed into crumbs. Carbohydrate.

Breaded breast of lamb★★/*Epigramme d'agneau*: high part of the cutlet. Red meat.

Breaded fish/*Poisson pané*: fish with white flesh coated with breadcrumbs.

Breaded knuckle of ham/*Jambonneau pané*: part of the leg above the knee breaded with wheat breadcrumbs. Cooked meat.

Breaded meat★★/*Viande panée*: meat coated with breadcrumbs.
Note: many commercially prepared foods are high in salt: prepare it yourself without salt and with authorized foods.

Breadfruit★★/*Fruit à pain*: fruit from the breadfruit tree.
Note: consume it immediately after the meal.

Bread with dried fruits/*Pain aux fruits secs*: bread enriched with dried fruits. Carbohydrate.

Bread with grains/*Pain aux graines*: wholewheat bread with crushed or whole grains. Carbohydrate.

Breakfast cookie/*Biscuit pour petit-déjeuner*: cookie adapted to breakfast, rich in cereals. Carbohydrate.

Breakfast sugary extruded cereal/*Céréale extrudée sucrée pour petit-déjeuner*: swelled cereal coated in sugar, honey, chocolat, etc. Carbohydrate.

Bream★★★/*Brème*: freshwater fish with white flesh.

Breckland thyme★★★/*Serpolet*: plant used as a condiment.

Brewer's yeast★★★/*Levure de bière*: unicellular microscopic mushrooms.

Brick cheese: pasteurised cow's milk cheese. Dairy product.

Brie cheese/*Brie*: soft aged cow's milk cheese with bloomy rind. Dairy product.

Brill★★★/*Barbue*: saltwater fish with white flesh.

Brillat-savarin cheese/*Brillat-savarin*: soft raw cow's milk cheese with bloomy rind. Triple cream cheese. Dairy product.

Brined anchovy/*Anchois en saumure*: anchovy fillet preserved in salt.

Brioche/*Brioche*: puffy pastry made of flour, yeast, fats and eggs.

Brioche bread/*Pain brioché*: cf. "Brioche".

Brioche crispbread/*Biscotte briochée*: slice of brioche sandwich bread industrially toasted in the oven. Carbohydrate.

Brocciu/*Broccio*: goat or sheep milk cheese. Dairy product.

Broccoli★★★/*Chou brocoli*: cabbage from which we eat the central inflorescence.

Broccoli seed★★★/*Graine de chou brocoli*: broccoli seed eaten crushed or germinated.

Broth★★/*Bouillon*: light soup made by boiling meat and vegetables in water.
Note: many commercially prepared foods are high in salt: prepare it yourself without salt and with authorized foods.

Brouillade★★/*Brouillade*: dish made of scrambled eggs.
Note: many commercially prepared foods are high in salt: prepare it yourself without salt and with authorized foods.

Brousse★★/*Brousse*: whey cheese made of goat, sheep or cow's milk very similar to ricotta. Dairy product.

Brown butter★★/*Beurre noisette*: butter heated until brown in a pan.
Note: no salted butter.

Brownie/*Brownie*: small chocolate cake with walnuts.

Brown mustard with cabbage leaf★★★/*Moutarde de Chine à feuille de chou*: vegetable plant from which we eat the leaves. Green vegetable.

Brown rice pasta/*Pâte alimentaire de riz brun*: cf. "Whole-grain rice pasta".

Brown sugar/*Sucre roux*: cane sugar which kept its impurities.

Brussel sprouts★★★/*Chou de Bruxelles*: vegetable plant from which we only eat the flower heads on the main stem.

Buckling/*Hareng saur*: salted herring smoked thanks to smoke.

Buckwheat bulgur★★★/*Boulgour de sarrasin*: sieved and crushed buckwheat steamed or cooked in water. Carbohydrate. Gluten-free.

Buckwheat cornflakes/*Corn flakes de sarrasin*: grilled flakes made of sieved buckwheat flakes. Carbohydrate. Gluten-free.

Buckwheat cream★★★/*Crème de sarrasin*: more or less liquid cream made of buckwheat milk, substitute to crème fraîche.

Buckwheat flake★★★/*Flocon de sarrasin*: small portion of dehydrated buckwheat. Carbohydrate.

Buckwheat milk★★/*Lait de sarrasin*: plant milk from buckwheat. Lactose-free.
Note: do not consume it sweetened.

Buckwheat milk cream dessert/*Crème dessert au lait de sarrasin*: vegetable dessert made of buckwheat milk, sugar and eggs.

Buckwheat pancake★★/*Galette*: flat, thin and round dish made of buckwheat flour, eggs and milk cooked in a frying pan. Carbohydrate. Gluten-free.
Note: many commercially prepared foods are high in salt: prepare it yourself without salt and with authorized foods.

Buckwheat pasta★★★/*Pâte alimentaire de sarrasin*: mix to be cooked made of refined buckwheat flour. Carbohydrate.

Buffalo/*Buffle*: cf. "Beef (meat)".

Bulgur★★★/*Boulgour*: sieved and crushed wheat steamed or cooked in water. Carbohydrate.

Bun/*Bun*: small round and puffy white bread. Carbohydrate.

Burger/*Burger*: round sandwich used as a staple in fast food restaurants. Carbohydrate.

Burger sauce/*Sauce burger*: sauce mainly made of vegetable oil, flavors, sugar and tomato purée.

Buttermilk★★★/*Babeurre*: liquid residue obtained after churning butter out of cream.

Button mangosteen in light syrup★/*Mangoustan au sirop léger*: poached button mangosteen preserved in more or less sugary water. Exotic fruit.

Button mangosteen in syrup/*Mangoustan au sirop*: poached button mangosteen preserved in very sugary water. Exotic fruit.

Button mangosteen juice/*Jus de mangoustan*: juice made of the pressing of button mangosteens. Exotic fruit.

Button mushroom★★★/*Champignon de Paris*: small edible white mushroom.
Note: do not eat canned vegetables (unless low in salt).

Buxton blue: raw or pasteurised cow's milk cheese. Dairy product.

C

Cabbage (red, white, green)★★★/*Chou pommé (rouge, blanc, vert)*: vegetable plant from which we eat the leaves.
Note: do not eat canned vegetables (unless low in salt).

Cachou/*Cachou*: aromatic pastille flavored with areca nut.

Caerphilly cheese: raw or pasteurised cow's milk cheese. Dairy product.

Café liégeois/*Liégeois (café)*: coffee ice cream coated with whipped cream.

Cake/*Gâteau*: pastry made of a batter used alone or with a cream, fruits...

Calf's head★★★/*Tête de veau*: calf's head eaten boiled. Offal.

Calisson/*Calisson*: candy in a diamond shape made of almonds and which top is frosted.

Camelina sativa oil★★★/*Huile de cameline*: fatty substance made of camelina sativa.

Camembert/*Camembert*: aged soft cow's milk cheese with bloomy rind. Dairy product.

Canapé/*Canapé*: small slice of sandwich bread on which various mixtures are spread. Carbohydrate.

Cancoillotte/*Cancoillotte*: low-fat melted cow's milk cheese. Dairy product.

Candied apple/*Pomme confite*: apple preserved thanks to the replacement of its water by sugar.

Candied apricot/*Abricot confit*: fresh apricot greatly enriched with sugar.

Candied aronia/*Aronia confite*: aronia preserved thanks to the replacement of its water by sugar.

Candied azerole/*Azerole confite*: azerole preserved thanks to the replacement of its water by sugar.

Candied banana/*Banane confite*: banana preserved thanks to the replacement of its water by sugar. Exotic fruit.

Candied blackberry/*Mûre confite*: blackberry preserved thanks to the replacement of its water by sugar.

Candied blackcurrant/*Cassis confit*: blackcurrant berry preserved thanks to the replacement of its water by sugar.

Candied blueberry/*Myrtille confite*: blueberry preserved thanks to the replacement of its water by sugar.

Candied button mangosteen/*Mangoustan confit*: button mangosteen preserved thanks to the replacement of its water by sugar. Exotic fruit.

Candied carambola/*Carambole confite*: carambola preserved thanks to the replacement of its water by sugar. Exotic fruit.

Candied cherimoya/*Anone confite*: cherimoya preserved thanks to the replacement of its water by sugar. Exotic fruit.

Candied cherry/*Cerise confite*: cherry preserved thanks to the replacement of its water by sugar.

Candied chestnut/*Marron glacé*: chestnut candied in sugar and iced with syrup.

Candied chili pepper in vinegar★★★/*Piment confit au vinaigre*: chili pepper preserved in vinegar. Green vegetable.
Note: only if it's salt-free or low-salt.

Candied clementine/*Clémentine confite*: clementine preserved thanks to the replacement of its water by sugar.

Candied coconut/*Noix de coco confite*: coconut pulp preserved thanks to the replacement of its water by sugar. Exotic fruit.

Candied cocoplum/*Icaque confit*: cocoplum preserved thanks to the replacement of its water by sugar. Exotic fruit.

Candied cranberry/*Canneberge confite*: cranberry preserved thanks to the replacement of its water by sugar.

Candied date/*Datte confite*: date preserved thanks to the replacement of its water by sugar. Exotic fruit.

Candied fig/*Figue confite*: fig preserved thanks to the replacement of its water by sugar.

Candied fruit/*Fruit confit*: fruit cooked in sugar syrup before being slowly dried.

Candied ginger/*Gingembre confit*: slice of ginger cooked and candied in sugar syrup.

Candied goji berry/*Baie de goji confite*: small red fruit eaten after being greatly enriched in sugar.

Candied grape/*Raisin confit*: grape preserved thanks to the replacement of its water by sugar.

Candied grapefruit/*Pamplemousse confit*: grapefruit preserved thanks to the replacement of its water by sugar.

Candied guava/*Goyave confite*: guava preserved thanks to the replacement of its water by sugar. Exotic fruit.

Candied jujube/Jujube confite: jujube preserved thanks to the replacement of its water by sugar. Exotic fruit.

Candied kaki/*Kaki confit*: kaki preserved thanks to the replacement of its water by sugar.

Candied kiwi/*Kiwi confit*: kiwi preserved thanks to the replacement of its water by sugar.

Candied kumquat/*Kumquat confit*: kumquat preserved thanks to the replacement of its water by sugar.

Candied lemon/*Citron confit*: lemon preserved thanks to the replacement of its water by sugar.

Candied longan/*Longane confite*: longan preserved thanks to the replacement of its water by sugar. Exotic fruit.

Candied lychee/*Litchi confit*: lychee preserved thanks to the replacement of its water by sugar. Exotic fruit.

Candied Malay rose apple/*Jambose confite*: Malay rose apple preserved thanks to the replacement of its water by sugar. Exotic fruit.

Candied mandarin/*Mandarine confite*: mandarin preserved thanks to the replacement of its water by sugar.

Candied mango/*Mangue confite*: mango preserved thanks to the replacement of its water by sugar. Exotic fruit.

Candied meat/*Viande confite*: cooked meat preserved in is fat.

Candied medlar/*Nèfle confite*: medlar preserved thanks to the replacement of its water by sugar.

Candied melon/*Melon confit*: melon preserved thanks to the replacement of its water by sugar.

Candied mirabelle plum/*Mirabelle confite*: mirabelle plum preserved thanks to the replacement of its water by sugar.

Candied mombins/*Mombin confit*: mombins preserved thanks to the replacement of its water by sugar. Exotic fruit.

Candied mulberries/*Mulberries confite*: mulberries preserved thanks to the replacement of its water by sugar.

Candied myrciaria/*Camu-camu confite*: myrciaria preserved thanks to the replacement of its water by sugar. Exotic fruit.

Candied orange/*Orange confite*: orange preserved thanks to the replacement of its water by sugar.

Candied papaya/*Papaye confite*: papaya preserved thanks to the replacement of its water by sugar. Exotic fruit.

Candied passion fruit/*Grenadille confite*: passion fruit preserved thanks to the replacement of its water by sugar. Exotic fruit.

Candied peach/*Pêche confite*: peach preserved thanks to the replacement of its water by sugar.

Candied pear/*Poire confite*: pear preserved thanks to the replacement of its water by sugar.

Candied physalis/*Physalis confite*: physalis preserved thanks to the replacement of its water by sugar. Exotic fruit.

Candied pineapple/*Ananas confit*: pineapple preserved thanks to the replacement of its water by sugar. Exotic fruit.

Candied plum/*Prune confite*: plum preserved thanks to the replacement of its water by sugar.

Candied quince/*Coing confit*: quince preserved thanks to the replacement of its water by sugar.

Candied rambutan/*Ramboutan confit*: rambutan preserved thanks to the replacement of its water by sugar. Exotic fruit.

Candied raspberry/*Framboise confite*: raspberry preserved thanks to the replacement of its water by sugar.

Candied redcurrant/*Groseille confite*: redcurrant preserved thanks to the replacement of its water by sugar.

Candied salak/*Salacca confit*: salak preserved thanks to the replacement of its water by sugar. Exotic fruit.

Candied sapodilla/*Sapotille confite*: sapodilla fruit preserved thanks to the replacement of its water by sugar. Exotic fruit.

Candied sloe/*Prunelle confite*: sloe preserved thanks to the replacement of its water by sugar.

Candied sorb/*Sorbe confite*: sorb preserved thanks to the replacement of its water by sugar.

Candied strawberry/*Fraise confite*: strawberry preserved thanks to the replacement of its water by sugar.

Candied tamarind fruit/*Tamarin confit*: tamarind fruit preserved thanks to the replacement of its water by sugar. Exotic fruit.

Candied vegetable★★/*Légume confit*: green vegetable preserved in vinegar.
Note: many commercially prepared foods are high in salt: prepare it yourself without salt and with authorized foods.

Candied watermelon
- Carambola in light syrup

Candied watermelon/*Pastèque confite*: watermelon preserved thanks to the replacement of its water by sugar.

Candy/*Bonbon*: confection only made of sugar and flavor.

Candy cane/*Sucre d'orge*: stick of flavored and cooked sugar. Fast-acting sugar.

Cannellonis/*Cannelloni*: wheat pasta rolled in the shape of a cylinder and stuffed with stuffing. Carbohydrate.

Canola oil★★★/*Huile de colza*: fatty substance made of canola.

Cantal cheese/*Cantal*: firm aged raw cow's milk cheese. Dairy product.

Cape gooseberry: cf. "Physalis peruviana".

Capelin★★★/*Capelan*: saltwater fish with white flesh.

Caper/*Câpre*: condiment. Flower bud from the caper bush candied in vinegar.

Capocollo/*Coppa*: cooked meat made of boned salted and smoked spare rib.

Capon★★★/*Chapon*: castrated cockerel. Poultry.

Cappuccino★★★/*Cappuccino*: foaming coffee with milk.
Note: do not drink it sweetened.

Capricious cheese: pasteurised goat's milk cheese. Dairy product.

Carambola in light syrup★/*Carambole au sirop léger*: poached carambola preserved in more or less sugary water. Exotic fruit.

Carambola in syrup/*Carambole au sirop*: poached carambola preserved in very sugary water. Exotic fruit.

Caramel(1)/*Caramel(1)*: product made from the action of the heat on sugar mixed with a little bit of water.

Caramel(2)/*Caramel(2)*: candy made of sugar and fats (cream, milk, butter...)

Caraway fruit★★★/*Carvi*: aromatic fruit from the caraway (plain plant).

Carbohydrate/*Féculent*: food more or less rich in starch such as potatoes, dry beans (beans from Soissons, cranberry beans, navy beans, kidney beans, lentils, split peas, flageolets, etc.), pasta, rice, quinoa, bread, grains (wheat, barley, rye, oats, etc.) and their equivalents: bulgur, semolina, etc. flours (see various flours in the previous pages), starches (see above), cassava, sweet potatoes, fava beans, plantains, etc. (See each carbohydrate separately in this book).

Carbonara sauce/*Sauce carbonara*: sauce made of crème fraîche, parmesan cheese, egg yolks and aromatic herbs.

Cardoon★★★/*Cardon*: vegetable plant from which we eat the plump part of the leaves. Green vegetable.
Note: do not eat canned vegetables (unless low in salt).

Caribbean reef octopus/*Chatrou*: small edible octopus.

Carob powder★★★/*Poudre de caroube*: instant drink made of carob powder.
Note: do not drink it sweetened.

Carob seeds flour★★★/*Farine de graines de caroube*: powder made of carob seeds milling. Gluten-free.

Carp★★★/*Carpe*: freshwater fish with white flesh.

Carré de l'Est/*Carré de l'Est*: soft cow's milk cheese with bloomy rind. Dairy product.

Carrot★★★/*Carotte*: vegetable plant grown for its edible root. Green vegetable.
Note: do not eat canned vegetables (unless low in salt).

Carrot juice/*Jus de carotte*: juice made of the pressing of carrots.

Carrots chips/*Chips de carottes*: very thinly cut carrots, fried and salted.

Carrot seed★★★/*Graine de carotte*: carrot seed eaten crushed or germinated.

Cashew milk★★/*Lait de noix de cajou*: plant milk from cashews. Lactose-free.
Note: do not consume it sweetened.

Cashew nut★★★/*Noix de cajou*: oleaginous seed from the cashew tree.
Note: do not consume cashew nut salted.

Cashew nut cream★★★/*Crème de noix de cajou*: more or less liquid cream made of cashew nut milk, substitute to crème fraîche.

Cashew nut milk cream dessert/*Crème dessert au lait de noix de cajou*: vegetable dessert made of cashew nut milk, sugar and eggs. Dairy product.

Cashew purée★★★/*Purée de noix de cajou*: mashed cashews to spread.

Cassava/*Manioc*: cf. "Tapioca".

Cassava flake★★★/*Flocon de manioc*: small portion of dehydrated cassava. Carbohydrate. Gluten-free.

Cassava flour/*Farine de manioc*: cf. "Tapioca". Carbohydrate.

Cassava starch/*Fécule de manioc*: cf. "Tapioca". Carbohydrate.

Cassoulet★★/*Cassoulet*: stew made of navy beans and goose confit, confit of duck, preserve of sheep or preserve of pork.
Note: many commercially prepared foods are high in salt: prepare it yourself without salt and with authorized foods.

Castor oil★★★/*Huile de ricin*: fatty substance made of castor seeds.

Catfish★★★/*Poisson-chat*: freshwater fish with white flesh.

Cauliflower★★★/*Chou-fleur*: cabbage from which we eat the central inflorescence.
Note: do not eat canned vegetables (unless low in salt).

Caviar/*Caviar*: salt-cured roe.

Celeriac/*Céleri-rave*: vegetable plant, kind of celery from which we eat the plump base. Green vegetable.

Celery★★/*Céleri à couper*: vegetable plant from which we eat the petiole. Green vegetable.
Note: do not eat canned vegetables (unless low in salt).

Celery juice/*Jus de céleri*: juice made of the pressing of celeries.

Celery salt/*Sel de céleri*: celery in powder.

Celery seed★★★/*Graine de céleri*: celery seed eaten crushed or germinated.

Celery stick★★/*Céleri branche*: vegetable plant from which we eat the petioles. Green vegetable.
Note: do not eat canned vegetables (unless low in salt).

Cereal bar/*Barre de céréales*: very sugary bar made of various cereals.

Cereal crispbread/*Biscotte aux céréales*: cf. "Wholegrain crispbread". Carbohydrate.

Cereals/*Céréales*: wheat, millet, oats, barley, rye, rice, corn, etc. For each cereal, see their own denomination. Carbohydrate.

Cervelas/*Cervelas*: cooked saucisson, cooked meat.

Chabichou/*Chabichou*: aged goat milk cheese. Dairy product.

Chaerophyllum bulbosum★★★/*Cerfeuil tubéreux*: kind of chervil from which we eat the root. Green vegetable.
Note: do not eat canned vegetables (unless low in salt).

Champagne/*Champagne*: sparkling white wine.

Chaource cheese/*Chaource*: soft cow's milk cheese with bloomy rind. Dairy product.

Chard/*Bette*: vegetable plant from which we eat the lines and leaves. Green vegetable.

Chateaubriand★★/*Chateaubriand*: thick slice of grilled or stir fried beef fillet. Red meat.

Chayote★★★/*Chayote*: fruit grown in warm countries and which has the same shape as a big green pear. Exotic fruit.

Cheddar/*Cheddar*: hard cow's milk cheese. Dairy product.

Cheese★/*Fromage*: food produced thanks to the milk coagulation, the straining of the curds you get and potentially maturing. Dairy product.
Note: almost all cheeses are too salty.

Cheeseburger/*Cheeseburger*: hamburger with aged cheese.

Cheese gnocchi/*Gnocchi au fromage*: ball made of wheat semolina and potatoes enriched with cheese. Carbohydrate.

Cheese ravioli/*Ravioli de fromage*: small square of pasta stuffed with various cheese before being poached. Carbohydrate.

Cheese with cereals/*Fromage aux céréales*: aged cheese with various cereals and/or cereal grains.

Cheese with dried fruits/*Fromage aux fruits secs*: aged cheese with various dried fruits.

Cheese with grains/*Fromage aux graines*: aged cheese with various grains.

Cheese with nuts/*Fromage aux noix*: aged cheese with more or less crushed nuts.

Cheese with parsley in its rind/*Fromage à pâte persillée*: blue cheese, fourme d'Ambert, gorgonzola, bleu du Vercors-Sassenage, stilton cheese... Dairy product.

Cheese with pepper/*Fromage au poivre*: aged cheese which surface is covered with peppercorns.

Cherimoya in light syrup★/*Anone au sirop léger*: poached cherimoya preserved in more or less sugary water. Exotic fruit.

Cherimoya in syrup/*Anone au sirop*: poached cherimoya preserved in very sugary water. Exotic fruit.

Cherry in light syrup
- Chestnut milk cream dessert

Cherry in light syrup★/*Cerise au sirop léger*: poached cherry preserved in more or less sugary water.

Cherry in syrup/*Cerise au sirop*: poached cherry preserved in very sugary water.

Cherry juice/*Jus de cerise*: juice made of the pressing of cherries.

Chervil★★★/*Cerfeuil*: leaf of an aromatic plant used as a condiment. Green vegetable.
Note: do not eat canned vegetables (unless low in salt).

Cheshire cheese/*Chester*: hard cow's milk cheese with raw or pasteurized milk. Dairy product.

Chestnut★★★/*Châtaigne*: fruit from the sweet chestnut tree, rich in starch. Carbohydrate.
Note: do not eat canned chestnut (unless low in salt).

Chestnut cornflakes/*Corn flakes de châtaigne*: grilled flakes made of chestnut flour. Carbohydrate. Gluten-free.

Chestnut cream/*Crème de châtaigne*: chestnut spread.

Chestnut flake/*Flocon de châtaigne*: small portion of dehydrated extruded chestnut. Carbohydrate. Gluten-free.

Chestnut flour★★★/*Farine de châtaigne*: powder made of chestnut milling. Carbohydrate. Gluten-free.

Chestnut milk★★/*Lait de châtaigne*: plant milk from chestnuts. Lactose-free.
Note: do not consume it sweetened.

Chestnut milk cream dessert/*Crème dessert au lait de châtaigne*: vegetable dessert made of chestnut milk, sugar and eggs. Dairy product.

Chestnut pasta★★★/*Pâte alimentaire de châtaigne*: mix to be cooked made of chestnut flour. Carbohydrate. Gluten-free.

Chestnut purée★★★/*Purée de châtaigne*: mashed chestnuts to spread.

Chewing gum★★/*Chewing-gum*: substance designed to be chewed.

Chia flour★★★/*Farine de chia*: powder from chia seeds milling. Gluten-free.

Chia seed★★★/*Graine de chia*: chia seed eaten crushed.

Chicken★★★/*Poulet*: baby of the hen, killed before being an adult. Poultry.

Chicken egg★★★/*Œuf de poule*: edible product from the egg-laying of the chicken.

Chicken ham/*Jambon de poulet*: chicken flesh turned into ham before being cut in thin slices. Cooked meat.

Chicken liver confit/*Confit de foie de volaille*: chicken livers cooked and preserved in their cooking fats.

Chicken nuggets/*Nuggets de poulet*: breaded chicken breast pieces eaten fried.

Chicken rillettes/*Rillettes de poulet*: cooked meat made of chicken meat cooked in its fat.

Chickling vetch: cf. "Lathyrus sativus".

Chickpea★★★/*Pois chiche*: big grey-yellow pea. Carbohydrate. Gluten-free.

Chickpea flake★★★/***Flocon de pois chiches***: small portion of dehydrated chickpea flakes. Carbohydrate. Gluten-free.

Chickpea flour★★★/***Farine de pois chiche***: powder made of chickpea milling. Carbohydrate. Gluten-free.

Chickpea pasta★★★/***Pâte alimentaire de pois chiche***: mix to be cooked made of chickpea flour. Carbohydrate. Gluten-free.

Chicory(1)★★★/***Chicorée(1)***: escarole... Kind of Greek salad. Green vegetable.

Chicory(2)/*Chicorée(2)*: cf. "Chicory coffee".

Chicory coffee/*Café chicorée*: sour chicory with big roots grown as coffee ersatz.

Chicory seed★★★/***Graine de chicorée***: chicory seed eaten crushed or germinated.

Chili con carne★★/***Chili con carné***: Mexican spicy dish made of kidney beans and ground meat. Red meat.
Note: many commercially prepared foods are high in salt: prepare it yourself without salt and with authorized foods.

Chili pepper pâté/Pâte de piment: cf. "Fresh chili pepper".

Chili pepper purée/*Purée de piment*: cf. "Chili pepper". Green vegetable.

Chinese artichoke: cf. "Stachys affinis".

Chinese cabbage★★★/***Chou chinois***: kind of two cabbages: Napa cabbage and pak choi.
Note: do not eat canned vegetables (unless low in salt).

Chinese noodles of "..."/*Nouille chinoise de "..."*: cf. "Pasta of "..."

Chipolata/*Chipolata*: thin pork sausage. Cooked meat.

Chives★★★/*Ciboulette*: plant from which we eat the hollow and cylindrical leaves.

Chocolate balls/*Crotte de chocolat*: chocolate candy, confection.

Chocolate bar/*Barre chocolatée*: candy made of chocolate and sugar and/or fruits and/or cereals, etc.

Chocolate chip cookie/*Cookie*: small cookie with chocolate, dried fruit, etc. chips.

Chocolate mousse/*Mousse au chocolat*: dessert made of whipped egg whites, chocolate and sugar.

Chocolate spread/*Pâte chocolatée à tartiner*: very sugary and fat mix of chocolate and crushed hazelnuts.

Chokecherry juice/*Jus de baie d'aronia*: juice made of the pressing of chokecherries.

Chorizo/*Chorizo*: half-dried saucisson seasoned with red chili pepper. Cooked meat.

Chouquette/*Chouquette*: small choux bun covered with pieces of sugar.

Choux pastry/*Pâte à choux*: batter made of butter, flour and eggs.

Chub★★★/*Chevaine*: freshwater fish with white flesh.

Chuck steak★★/*Paleron de bœuf*: piece of beef to simmer or to boil. Red meat.

Chufa sedge milk★★/*Lait de horchata de chufa*: sweetened beverage made from chuff sedge tubers. Lactose-free.
Note: do not consume it sweetened.

Chutney★★/*Chutney*: sweet and sour condiment made of vegetables or fruits cooked with vinegar, spices and sugar.
Note: many commercially prepared foods are high in salt: prepare it yourself without salt and with authorized foods.

Cider★/*Cidre*: alcoholic beverage obtained thanks to the apple juice fermentation.
Note: do not drink alcoholic beverage, however no problem if it's cooked.

Cilantro★★★/*Coriandre*: aromatic plant used as a condiment. Green vegetable.

Cilantro seed★★★/*Graine de coriandre*: cilantro seed eaten crushed or germinated.

Cinnamon★★★/*Cannelle*: bark of the cinnamon tree used as seasoning.

Clafoutis★★/*Clafoutis*: cake baked in the oven made of a mixture of batter and fruits.
Note: many commercially prepared foods are high in salt: prepare it yourself without salt and sugar and with authorized foods.

Clam/*Praire*: edible saltwater mollusk.

Claytonia perfoliata★★★/*Claytone de Cuba*: vegetable plant you eat as a whole.

Clementine in light syrup★/*Clémentine au sirop léger*: poached clementine preserved in more or less sugary water.

Clementine in syrup/*Clémentine au sirop*: poached clementine preserved in very sugary water.

Clementine juice/*Jus de clémentine*: juice made of the pressing of clementines.

Clove★★★/*Clou de girofle*: fruit from the clove tree used as a spice.

Coalfish★★★/*Goberge*: saltwater fish white white flesh.

Cochlearia★★★/*Cochléaire*: edible plant which grows in damp places. Green vegetable.

Cockle/*Coque*: edible sea mollusk.

Cocktail/*Cocktail*: alcoholic beverage with fruits, fruit juice, syrup, etc.

Cocktail sausage/*Saucisse cocktail*: small pork sausage with a smoky taste. Cooked meat.

Cocoa★★★/*Cacao*: seed of the cocoa tree used to make chocolate.

Cocoa butter★★★/*Beurre de cacao*: fat extracted from the cocoa.

Cocoa powder/*Cacao en poudre*: mix of cocoa powder and sugar.

Cocoa powder without sugar★★★/*Cacao en poudre non sucré*: cocoa powder without added sugar.

Coconut★★★/*Noix de coco*: fruit from the coconut palm. Exotic fruit.

Coconut cream★★★/*Crème de coco*: more or less liquid cream made of coconut milk, substitute to crème fraîche.

Coconut flour★★★/*Farine de coco*: powder from coconut pulp milling. Gluten-free.

Coconut flower sugar★/*Sucre de fleur de coco*: sugar from palm sap. Fast-acting sugar.

Coconut flower syrup/*Sirop de fleur de coco*: sugary syrup made from the palm sap.

Coconut milk★★★/*Lait de coco*: plant milk from coconuts. Lactose-free.

Coconut milk cream dessert/*Crème dessert au lait de coco*: vegetable dessert made of coconut milk, sugar and eggs. Dairy product.

Coconut milk yogurt/*Yaourt au lait de coco*: coconut milk fermented thanks to lactic acid bacteria, sweetened or not. Dairy product. Lactose-free.

Coconut oil★★★/*Huile de coco*: fatty substance made of coconut.

Coconut powdered sugar★/*Sucre glace de coco*: coconut flower sugar in extremely thin powder. Fast-acting sugar.

Coconut purée★★★/*Purée de coco*: mashed coconut pulp to spread.

Coconut rock cake/*Congolais*: small coconut cake.

Coconut water★★★/*Eau de coco*: water from the coconut.

Cocoplum in light syrup★/*Icaque au sirop léger*: poached cocoplum preserved in more or less sugary water. Exotic fruit.

Cocoplum in syrup/*Icaque au sirop*: poached cocoplum preserved in very sugary water. Exotic fruit.

Cod/*Morue*: saltwater fish with white flesh.

Cod liver/*Foie de morue*: cod liver in oil sold in can. Offal.

Cod liver oil★★★/*Huile de foie de morue*: fatty substance made of cod liver.

Coffee★★★/*Café*: seed of the coffee bush rich in caffeine and drunk once roasted.
Note: do not drink soluble coffee and do not drink it sweetened.

Cognac★/*Cognac*: brandy made of wine from the Cognac area in France.
Note: do not drink alcoholic beverage, however no problem if it's cooked.

Colby cheese: pasteurised cow's milk cheese. Dairy product.

Cold-pressed extra virgin olive oil★★★/*Huile d'olive extra vierge pressée à froid*: fatty substance made of very high nutritional quality olive.

Coley★★★/*Colin*: saltwater fish with white flesh.

Colombo★★★/*Colombo*: mix of spices made of garlic, cilantro, chili pepper, cinnamon, turmeric, etc.

Comber★★★/*Serran*: saltwater fish with white flesh.

Common dace★★★/*Vandoise*: freshwater fish with white flesh.

Common nase★★★/*Hotu*: freshwater fish with white flesh.

Common rudd★★★/*Rotengle*: freshwater fish with white flesh.

Common smooth-hound★★★/*Emissole*: small edible shark with white flesh.

Comté cheese/*Comté*: hard cow's milk. Dairy product.

Concentrate fruit juice/*Jus de fruit concentré*: reconstituted fruit juice made of fruit juice and water.

Confection/*Confiserie*: various candies.

Confit of duck/*Confit de canard*: duck cooked and preserved in its fat.

Conger★★★/*Congre*: fatty saltwater fish.

Consommé★★/*Consommé*: meat stock.
Note: many commercially prepared foods are high in salt: prepare it yourself without salt and with authorized foods.

Cooked meat/*Charcuterie*: product made of cooked or raw salted pork meat. See each cooked meat separately.

Cookie without added sugar/*Biscuit sans sucre ajouté*: sweetened cookie without added sugar containing only the sugar that is naturally present in the ingredients. Carbohydrate.

Cooking oil★★★/*Huile de friture*: mix of vegetable oils especially made for frying.

Copra oil★★★/*Huile de coprah*: fatty substance made of copra.

Coquetdale cheese: cow's milk cheese with pasteurized milk. Dairy product.

Coregonus albula★★★/*Corégone*: freshwater fish with white flesh.

Core oil★★★/*Huile de noyaux*: fatty substance made of various fruit cores.

Corn bran★★★/*Son de maïs*: residue of corn milling.

Corn cornflakes/*Corn flakes de maïs*: grilled flakes made of sieved corn flakes. Carbohydrate. Gluten-free.

Corned-beef/*Corned beef*: beef meat preserved and salted. Red meat.

Corn flake★★★/*Flocon de maïs*: small portion of dehydrated corn. Carbohydrate. Gluten-free.

Corn flour★★★/*Farine de maïs*: powder made of not whole-grain corn milling. Carbohydrate. Gluten-free.

Corn oil★★★/*Huile de maïs*: fatty substance made of corn.

Corn pasta★★★/*Pâte alimentaire de maïs*: mix to be cooked made of refined corn flour. Carbohydrate. Gluten-free.

Cornstarch★★★/*Fécule de maïs*: not whole-grain corn flour. Carbohydrate.

Corn syrup/*Sirop de maïs*: sweetener made of corn starch.

Cottage cheese: pasteurised cow's milk cheese. Dairy product.

Cotignac/*Cotignac*: very sugary quince jelly.

Cotton oil★★★/*Huile de coton*: fatty substance made of cotton.

Coulis★★/*Coulis*: sauce made of various food substances transformed into purée.
Note: many commercially prepared foods are high in salt and/or in sugar so prepare it yourself without salt and sugar and with authorized foods.

Coulommiers cheese/*Coulommiers*: soft cow's milk cheese with bloomy rind. Dairy product.

Country-style pâté/*Pâté de campagne*: ground meat made of pork meat, fat and poultry livers.

Couscous★/*Couscous*: North African dish made of hard wheat semolina, meat, fish and various vegetables.
Note: many commercially prepared foods are high in salt: prepare it yourself without salt and with authorized foods.

Cowpea★★★/*Dolique*: plant looking like a bean growing in tropical regions. Green vegetable.

Cow's milk cheese★/*Fromage de vache*: cheese made of cow's milk. Dairy product.
Note: almost all cheeses are too salty.

Cow's milk cottage cheese★★★/*Faisselle au lait de vache*: fresh cheese made of cow's milk. Dairy product.

Cow's milk cream dessert/*Crème dessert au lait de vache*: dairy specialty or dessert made of cow's milk, sugar and eggs. Dairy product.

Cow's milk fromage blanc★★★/*Fromage blanc de vache*: fresh cheese made of cow's milk, a bit drained and not aged. Dairy product.

Cow's trotter★★★/*Pied de veau*: veal foot. Offal.

Crab/*Crabe*: sea crustacean you can find on the coastline or in freshwater.

Crab rillettes/*Rillettes de crabe*: cooked meat made of crab flesh cooked in vegetable oil.

Cracker/*Cracker*: small salted cookie for the aperitif. Carbohydrate.

Crambe★/*Crambe*: plant also called seakale. Green vegetable.

Cranberry in light syrup★/*Canneberge au sirop léger*: poached cranberry preserved in more or less sugary water.

Cranberry in syrup/*Canneberge au sirop*: poached cranberry preserved in very sugary water.

Cranberry juice/*Jus de cranberry*: juice made of the pressing of cranberries.

Crangon crangon/*Boucaud*: grey shrimp.

Crawfish/*Ecrevisse*: freshwater crustacean liked for its flesh.

Crayfish/*Langouste*: walking crustacean very appreciated for its flesh.

Crème aux œufs/*Crème aux œufs*: cf. "Cream dessert".

Crème bachique★★/*Crème bachique*: dessert made of eggs, sugar and rum.
Note: many commercially prepared foods are high in sugar, so prepare it yourself without sugar and with authorized foods.

Crème brûlée/*Crème brûlée*: cf. "Cream dessert with cow's milk".

Crème caramel★★/*Crème renversée*: dessert made of milk, sugar and whisked eggs cooked in a bain-marie and removed from the mold before being turned. Dairy product.
Note: many commercially prepared foods are high in sugar, so prepare it yourself without sugar and with authorized foods.

Crepe★★/*Crêpe*: thin layer of cooked batter made of eggs, milk and flour. Carbohydrate.
Note: many commercially prepared foods are high in salt and/or in sugar so prepare it yourself without salt and sugar and with authorized foods.

Crépinette/*Crépinette*: flat sausage. Cooked meat.

Crimson beebalm
- Crunchy barley slice of bread

Crimson beebalm★★★/*Monarde écarlate*: plant which leaves are used as an aromatic condiment.

Croissant/*Croissant*: viennoiserie pastry made of flour, butter and sugar.

Croque madame/*Croque-madame*: croque-monsieur with an egg on top.

Croque monsieur/*Croque-monsieur*: hot dish made of ham and cheese between two slices of sandwich bread.

Crottin de Chavignol/*Crottin de Chavignol*: small raw goat milk cheese. Dairy product.

Crouton/*Croûton*: small piece of fried white bread. Carbohydrate.

Crowdie: pasteurised cow's milk cheese. Dairy product.

Crucian carp★★★/*Cyprin*: freshwater fish with white flesh.

Crudité★★★/*Crudité*: green vegetable or fruit eaten raw.

Crumble/*Crumble*: dessert made of fruits covered with sweet shortcrust pastry and baked in the oven.

Crunchy amaranth slice of bread/*Tartine craquante amarante*: flat and light extruded slice of bread made of refined amaranth flour. Carbohydrate. Gluten-free.

Crunchy barley slice of bread/*Tartine craquante orge*: flat and light extruded slice of bread made of refined barley flour. Carbohydrate.

Crunchy buckwheat slice of bread/*Tartine craquante sarrasin*: flat and light extruded slice of bread made of refined buckwheat flour. Carbohydrate. Gluten-free.

Crunchy carob seed slice of bread/*Tartine craquante graine de caroube*: flat and light extruded slice of bread made of refined carob seed flour. Carbohydrate. Gluten-free.

Crunchy cassava slice of bread/*Tartine craquante manioc*: flat and light extruded slice of bread made of refined cassava flour. Carbohydrate. Gluten-free.

Crunchy chestnut slice of bread/*Tartine craquante châtaigne*: flat and light extruded slice of bread made of chestnut flour. Carbohydrate. Gluten-free.

Crunchy chia slice of bread/*Tartine craquante chia*: flat and light extruded slice of bread made of chia flour. Carbohydrate. Gluten-free.

Crunchy chickpea slice of bread/*Tartine craquante pois chiche*: flat and light extruded slice of bread made of chickpea flour. Carbohydrate. Gluten-free.

Crunchy coconut slice of bread/*Tartine craquante coco*: flat and light extruded slice of bread made of coconut flour. Carbohydrate. Gluten-free.

Crunchy corn slice of bread/*Tartine craquante maïs*: flat and light extruded slice of bread made of refined corn flour. Carbohydrate. Gluten-free.

Crunchy einkorn wheat slice of bread/*Tartine craquante petit épeautre*: flat and light extruded slice of bread made of refined einkorn wheat flour. Carbohydrate.

Crunchy findi slice of bread
- Crunchy oat slice of bread

Crunchy findi slice of bread/*Tartine craquante fonio*: flat and light extruded slice of bread made of refined findi flour. Carbohydrate. Gluten-free.

Crunchy flax slice of bread/*Tartine craquante lin*: flat and light extruded slice of bread made of flax flour. Carbohydrate. Gluten-free.

Crunchy gluten-free oat slice of bread/*Tartine craquante avoine sans gluten*: flat and light extruded slice of bread made of refined and gluten-free oat flour. Carbohydrate.

Crunchy khorasan wheat slice of bread/*Tartine craquante kamut*: flat and light extruded slice of bread made of refined khorasan wheat flour. Carbohydrate.

Crunchy lentil slice of bread/*Tartine craquante lentille*: flat and light extruded slice of bread made of lentil flour. Carbohydrate. Gluten-free.

Crunchy lupin slice of bread/*Tartine craquante lupin*: flat and light extruded slice of bread made of lupin flour. Carbohydrate. Gluten-free.

Crunchy millet slice of bread/*Tartine craquante millet*: flat and light extruded slice of bread made of refined millet flour. Carbohydrate. Gluten-free.

Crunchy multi-cereal slice of bread/*Tartine craquante multicéréale*: flat and light extruded slice of bread made of various cereals. Carbohydrate.

Crunchy nutsedge slice of bread/*Tartine craquante souchet*: flat and light extruded slice of bread made of nutsedge flour. Carbohydrate. Gluten-free.

Crunchy oat slice of bread/*Tartine craquante avoine*: flat and light extruded slice of bread made of refined oat flour. Carbohydrate.

Crunchy onion slice of bread/*Tartine craquante oignon*: flat and light extruded slice of bread made of onions. Carbohydrate.

Crunchy peanut slice of bread/*Tartine craquante arachide*: flat and light extruded slice of bread made of refined peanut flour. Carbohydrate. Gluten-free.

Crunchy quinoa slice of bread/*Tartine craquante quinoa*: flat and light extruded slice of bread made of refined quinoa flour. Carbohydrate. Gluten-free.

Crunchy rice slice of bread/*Tartine craquante riz*: flat and light extruded slice of bread made of refined rice flour. Carbohydrate. Gluten-free.

Crunchy rye slice of bread/*Tartine craquante seigle*: flat and light extruded slice of bread made of refined rye flour. Carbohydrate.

Crunchy sesame slice of bread/*Tartine craquante sésame*: flat and light extruded slice of bread made of sesame. Carbohydrate. Gluten-free.

Crunchy sorghum slice of bread/*Tartine craquante sorgho*: flat and light extruded slice of bread made of sorghum flour. Carbohydrate. Gluten-free.

Crunchy soybean slice of bread/*Tartine craquante soja*: flat and light extruded slice of bread made of refined soybean flour. Carbohydrate. Gluten-free.

Crunchy spelt slice of bread/*Tartine craquante épeautre*: flat and light extruded slice of bread made of refined spelt flour. Carbohydrate.

Crunchy squash seed slice of bread/*Tartine craquante pépin de courge*: flat and light extruded slice of bread made of squash seed flour. Carbohydrate. Gluten-free.

Crunchy sweet potato slice of bread
- Crunchy whole-grain findi slice of bread

Crunchy sweet potato slice of bread/*Tartine craquante patate douce*: flat and light extruded slice of bread made of sweet potato flour. Carbohydrate. Gluten-free.

Crunchy teff slice of bread/*Tartine craquante teff*: flat and light extruded slice of bread made of refined teff flour. Carbohydrate. Gluten-free.

Crunchy wheat slice of bread/*Tartine craquante froment*: flat and light extruded slice of bread made of refined tender wheat flour. Carbohydrate.

Crunchy whole-grain amaranth slice of bread/*Tartine craquante amarante complète*: flat and light extruded slice of bread made of whole-grain amaranth flour. Carbohydrate. Gluten-free.

Crunchy whole-grain barley slice of bread/*Tartine craquante orge complète*: flat and light extruded slice of bread made of whole-grain barley flour. Carbohydrate.

Crunchy whole-grain buckwheat slice of bread/*Tartine craquante sarrasin complète*: flat and light extruded slice of bread made of whole-grain buckwheat flour. Carbohydrate. Gluten-free.

Crunchy whole-grain corn slice of bread/*Tartine craquante maïs complète*: flat and light extruded slice of bread made of whole-grain corn flour. Carbohydrate. Gluten-free.

Crunchy whole-grain einkorn wheat slice of bread/*Tartine craquante petit épeautre complète*: flat and light extruded slice of bread made of whole-grain einkorn wheat flour. Carbohydrate.

Crunchy whole-grain findi slice of bread/*Tartine craquante fonio complète*: flat and light extruded slice of bread made of whole-grain findi flour. Carbohydrate. Gluten-free.

Crunchy whole-grain khorasan wheat slice of bread - Crunchy whole-grain spelt slice of bread

Crunchy whole-grain khorasan wheat slice of bread/*Tartine craquante kamut complète*: flat and light extruded slice of bread made of whole-grain khorasan wheat flour. Carbohydrate.

Crunchy whole-grain oat slice of bread/*Tartine craquante avoine complète*: flat and light extruded slice of bread made of whole-grain oat flour. Carbohydrate.

Crunchy whole-grain peanut slice of bread/*Tartine craquante arachide complète*: flat and light extruded slice of bread made of whole-grain peanut flour. Carbohydrate. Gluten-free.

Crunchy whole-grain quinoa slice of bread/*Tartine craquante quinoa complète*: flat and light extruded slice of bread made of whole-grain quinoa. Carbohydrate. Gluten-free.

Crunchy whole-grain rice slice of bread/*Tartine craquante riz complet*: flat and light extruded slice of bread made of whole-grain rice flour. Carbohydrate. Gluten-free.

Crunchy whole-grain rye slice of bread/*Tartine craquante seigle complète*: flat and light extruded slice of bread made of whole-grain rye flour. Carbohydrate.

Crunchy whole-grain soybean slice of bread/*Tartine craquante soja complète*: flat and light extruded slice of bread made of whole-grain soybean flour. Carbohydrate. Gluten-free.

Crunchy whole-grain spelt slice of bread/*Tartine craquante épeautre complète*: flat and light extruded slice of bread made of whole-grain spelt flour. Carbohydrate.

Crunchy whole-grain teff slice of bread
- Cube of low-salt chicken broth

Crunchy whole-grain teff slice of bread/*Tartine craquante teff complète*: flat and light extruded slice of bread made of whole-grain teff flour. Carbohydrate. Gluten-free.

Crunchy wholewheat slice of bread/*Tartine craquante blé complète*: flat and light extruded slice of bread made of wholewheat flour. Carbohydrate.

Crunchy yam slice of bread/*Tartine craquante igname*: flat and light extruded slice of bread made of refined yam flour. Carbohydrate. Gluten-free.

Crushed spelt/*Epeautre concassé*: cf. "Spelt bulgur".

Crustacean/*Crustacé*: crab, lobster, shrimp, etc.

Cube of beef broth/*Bouillon de bœuf en cube*: cube of dehydrated industrial beef broth.

Cube of beef stew broth/*Bouillon de pot-au-feu en cube*: cf. "Cube of beef broth".

Cube of chicken broth/*Bouillon de volaille en cube*: cube of dehydrated industrial chicken broth.

Cube of low-fat beef broth/*Bouillon de bœuf dégraissé en cube*: cube of low-fat and dehydrated industrial beef broth.

Cube of low-fat chicken broth/*Bouillon de volaille dégraissé en cube*: cube of low-fat and dehydrated industrial chicken broth.

Cube of low-fat vegetable broth/*Bouillon de légumes dégraissé en cube*: cube of low-fat and dehydrated industrial vegetable broth.

Cube of low-salt chicken broth★/*Bouillon de volaille allégé en sel en cube*: cube of light-sodium and dehydrated industrial chicken broth.

Cube of salt-free vegetable broth★★★/*Bouillon de légumes sans sel en cube*: cube of salt-free and dehydrated industrial vegetable broth.

Cube of vegetable broth/*Bouillon de légumes en cube*: cube of dehydrated industrial vegetable broth.

Cucumber★★★/*Concombre*: vegetable plant grown for its long fruit.

Cuidité★★★/*Cuidité*: green vegetable or fruit eaten cooked.
Note: do not eat canned vegetables (unless low in salt). Cook it without salt and sugar.

Cumin★★★/*Cumin*: spice.

Cumin seed★★★/*Graine de cumin*: cumin seed eaten crushed or germinated.

Cup cheese: melted cheese. Dairy product.

Curaçao/*Curaçao*: liqueur made of orange peel, sugar and eau de vie.

Curly endive (lettuce)★★★/*Frisée (laitue)*: lettuce with curly leaves eaten in salad. Green vegetable.

Curry★★★/*Curry*: mix of Indian spices.

Curuba★★/*Curuba*: exotic fruit from Asia.
Note: consume it immediately after the meal.

Custard(1)★★/*Crème anglaise*: cream with a base thickened on the heat and flavored with vanilla. Dairy product.
Note: many commercially prepared foods are high in sugar, so prepare it yourself without sugar and with authorized foods.

Custard(2)★★/*Crème pâtissière*: cream made of flour, eggs, milk and sugar. Dairy product.
Note: many commercially prepared foods are high in sugar, so prepare it yourself without sugar and with authorized foods.

Custard apple★★/*Chérimole*: fruit from the cherimoya. Exotic fruit.
Note: consume it immediately after the meal.

Cuttlefish/*Seiche*: saltwater mollusk close to the squid.

Cyclanthera★★★/*Cyclanthère*: young fruit preserved in vinegar.

Dab★★★/*Limande*: flat saltwater fish with white flesh.

Dandelion★★★/*Pissenlit*: plant from which we eat the young leaves in salad. Green vegetable.

Dandelion coffee★★★/*Café de pissenlit*: drink made of dried dandelion roots.
Note: do not drink it sweetened.

Dark chocolate★★/*Chocolat noir*: chocolate containing between 43 % and 100 % of cocoa and cocoa butter, the rest being mainly sugar.

Date honey/*Sirop de datte*: sugary syrup made of date extracts.

Date jelly/*Pâte de datte*: cf. "Dried date".

Daube★★/*Daube*: culinary technique consisting in braising beef with a base of red wine. Red meat.
Note: many commercially prepared foods are high in salt: prepare it yourself without salt and with authorized foods.

Dauphinois (gratin)/*Dauphinois (gratin)*: dish made of thin slices of grilled potatoes with milk, butter and cheese.

Decaffeinated coffee/*Café soluble décaféiné*: grains of dehydrated decaffeinated coffee.

Decaffeinated espresso★★★/*Expresso décaféiné*: caffeine-free express coffee.
Note: do not drink it sweetened.

Deer (meat)★★/*Daim (viande de)*: game from which we eat the meat. Red meat.

Dehydrated green vegetable soup/*Potage de légumes verts déshydraté*: dehydrated industrial soup.

Derby cheese: raw or pasteurised cow's milk cheese. Dairy product.

Dessert★★/*Entremets*: sugary dish which is not pastry. Dairy product.
Note: many commercially prepared foods are high in sugar, so prepare it yourself without sugar and with authorized foods.

Dessert wine/*Vin liquoreux*: white wine which contains more than 45 grams of sugar per liter.

Deviled egg★★/*Œuf mimosa*: egg cut in half, the egg yolk is removed and mixed with mayonnaise, before filling the hole in the white part of the egg with this mixture.
Note: consume it only with mayonnaise unsalted.

"Diet" extruded cereal/*Céréale extrudée "de régime"*: sugar-free and low-calorie swelled cereal. High glycemic index. Carbohydrate.

"Diet" salt★★★/*Sel "de régime"*: potassium chloride used to season dishes. Some diet salts offer one third of the total quantity of sodium chloride (standard table salt).
Note: ask your doctor if you can consume it!

Dill★★★/*Aneth*: aromatic umbellifer plant.

Dock★★★/*Patience*: vegetable plant from which we eat the leaves. Green vegetable.

Doe (meat)★★/*Biche (viande de)*: female deer. Red meat. Game.

Dog cockle/*Amande marin*: edible sea mollusk.

Dogfish★★★/*Roussette*: cartilaginous saltwater fish (small shark) with white flesh.

Donax/*Donax*: small edible sea mollusk.

Dorset blue vinney: raw cow's milk cheese. Dairy product.

Double cream cheese★/*Fromage double crème*: cheese containing between 60 and 75% of fats. Dairy product.
Note: almost all cheeses are too salty.

Dovedale cheese: pasteurised cow's milk cheese. Dairy product.

Double Gloucester: raw or pasteurised cow's milk cheese. Dairy product.

Dried apple/*Pomme séchée*: apple which went under a desiccation process under the sun.

Dried apricot/*Abricot sec*: fresh apricot dehydrated thanks to the action of the sun or that of the heat.

Dried aronia/*Aronia séchée*: aronia which went under a desiccation process under the sun.

Dried azerole/*Azerole séchée*: azerole which went under a desiccation process under the sun.

Dried banana/*Banane séchée*: banana which went under a desiccation process. Exotic fruit.

Dried bean★★★/*Haricot sec*: bean seed eaten ripe such as split peas, beans from Soissons, cranberry beans, navy beans, kidney beans, pinto beans, black turtle beans, lentils, chickpeas, flageolets, etc. Carbohydrate.

Dried blackberry/*Mûre séchée*: blackberry which went under a desiccation process under the sun.

Dried blackcurrant/*Cassis séché*: blackcurrant which went under a desiccation process under the sun.

Dried button mangosteen/*Mangoustan séché*: button mangosteen which went under a desiccation process under the sun. Exotic fruit.

Dried carambola/*Carambole séchée*: carambola which went under a desiccation process under the sun. Exotic fruit.

Dried cherimoya/*Anone séchée*: cherimoya which went under a desiccation process under the sun. Exotic fruit.

Dried cherry/*Cerise séchée*: cherry which went under a desiccation process under the sun.

Dried chili pepper★★★/*Piment sec*: chili pepper which went under a desiccation process under the sun. Green vegetable.

Dried clementine/*Clémentine séchée*: clementine which went under a desiccation process under the sun.

Dried coconut/*Noix de coco séchée*: coconut pulp fragment eaten after being completely desiccated. Exotic fruit.

Dried cranberry/*Canneberge séchée*: cranberry which went under a desiccation process under the sun.

Dried date/*Datte séchée*: fruit from the date palm which dried under the sun. Exotic fruit.

Dried fatty fish/*Poisson gras séché*: fatty fish which went under a desiccation process.

Dried fig/Figue séchée: fig which has been dried under the sun

Dried fruit/*Fruit sec*: fruit which went under a desiccation process under the sun.

Dried fruits breakfast cookie/*Biscuit pour petit-déjeuner aux fruits secs*: cookie with dried fruits adapted to breakfast. Carbohydrate.

Dried goji berry/*Baie de goji séchée*: small red fruit eaten after a complete desiccation process.

Dried grapefruit/*Pamplemousse séché*: grapefruit which went under a desiccation process under the sun.

Dried guava/*Goyave séchée*: guava which went under a desiccation process under the sun. Exotic fruit.

Dried jackfruit/*Jaque séché*: jackfruit which went under a desiccation process under the sun.

Dried jujube/*Jujube séchée*: jujube which went under a desiccation process under the sun. Exotic fruit.

Dried kaki/*Kaki séché*: kaki which went under a desiccation process under the sun.

Dried kiwi/*Kiwi séché*: kiwi which went under a desiccation process under the sun.

Dried kumquat/*Kumquat séché*: kumquat which went under a desiccation process under the sun.

Dried lean fish/*Poisson maigre séché*: lean fish which went under a desiccation process.

Dried legume★★★/*Légume sec*: legume seeds (lentils, navy beans, beans from Soissons, cranberry beans, favas, chickpeas, split peas, kidney beans, black turtle beans, lupins, mojette beans, common vetches, etc.) eaten ripe. Carbohydrate.

Dried lemon/*Citron séché*: lemon which went under a desiccation process under the sun.

Dried longan/*Longane séchée*: longan which went under a desiccation process under the sun. Exotic fruit.

Dried lychee/*Litchi séché*: lychee which went under a desiccation process under the sun. Exotic fruit.

Dried Malay rose apple/*Jambose séchée*: Malay rose apple which went under a desiccation process under the sun. Exotic fruit.

Dried mandarin/*Mandarine séchée*: mandarin which went under a desiccation process under the sun.

Dried mango/*Mangue séchée*: mango which went under a desiccation process under the sun. Exotic fruit.

Dried medlar/*Nèfle séchée*: medlar which went under a desiccation process under the sun.

Dried melon/*Melon séché*: melon which went under a desiccation process under the sun.

Dried mirabelle plum/*Mirabelle séchée*: mirabelle plum which went under a desiccation process under the sun.

Dried mombins/*Mombin séché* : mombins which went under a desiccation process under the sun. Exotic fruit.

Dried mulberries/*Mulberries séchée*: mulberries which went under a desiccation process under the sun.

Dried mushroom★★★/*Champignon séché*: fresh mushroom which went under a desiccation process. Green vegetable.

Dried myrciaria/*Camu-camu séchée*: myrciaria which went under a desiccation process under the sun. Exotic fruit.

Dried orange/*Orange séchée*: orange which went under a desiccation process under the sun.

Dried papaya/*Papaye séchée*: papaya which went under a desiccation process under the sun. Exotic fruit.

Dried passion fruit/*Fruit de la passion séché*: passion fruit which went under a desiccation process.

Dried peach/*Pêche séchée*: peach which went under a desiccation process under the sun.

Dried pear/*Poire séchée*: pear which went under a desiccation process under the sun.

Dried physalis/*Physalis séchée*: physalis which went under a desiccation process under the sun. Exotic fruit.

Dried pineapple/*Ananas séché*: pineapple which went under a desiccation process under the sun. Exotic fruit.

Dried pitaya/*Pitaya séchée*: pitaya which went under a desiccation process under the sun. Exotic fruit.

Dried pomegranate/*Grenade séchée*: pomegranate which went under a desiccation process under the sun. Exotic fruit.

Dried quince/*Coing séché*: quince which went under a desiccation process.

Dried rambutan/*Ramboutan séché*: rambutan which went under a desiccation process under the sun. Exotic fruit.

Dried raspberry/*Framboise séchée*: fresh raspberry which went under a desiccation process.

Dried redcurrant/*Groseille séchée*: redcurrant which went under a desiccation process under the sun.

Dried sapodilla fruit/Sapotille séchée: sapodilla fruit which went under a desiccation process under the sun. Exotic fruit.

Dried sloe/*Prunelle séchée*: sloe which went under a desiccation process under the sun.

Dried strawberry/*Fraise séchée*: fresh strawberry which went under a desiccation process.

Dried tamarind fruit/*Tamarin séché*: tamarind fruit which went under a desiccation process under the sun. Exotic fruit.

Dried watermelon/*Pastèque séchée*: watermelon which went under a desiccation process under the sun.

Dry-cured ham/*Jambon sec*: raw pork ham salted before being dried. Cooked meat.

Duck★★★/*Canard*: edible palmiped bird. Poultry.

Duck egg★★★/*Œuf de cane*: edible product from the egg-laying of the female duck.

Duck fat★★★/*Graisse de canard*: duck fat used to make confits.

Duck liver pâté/*Pâté de foie de canard*: minced duck liver cooked before being put in a baking pan. Cooked meat.

Dulse/*Dulce*: edible red seaweed.

Dunlop cheese: raw or pasteurised cow's milk cheese. Dairy product.

Durio zibethinus★★/*Durian*: exotic fruit from Asia.
Note: consume it immediately after the meal.

Duxelles★★/*Duxelles*: minced mixture of mushrooms, onions and shallots.
Note: many commercially prepared foods are high in salt: prepare it yourself without salt and with authorized foods.

E

Ear of corn★★★/*Epi de maïs*: young corn shoot considered as a green vegetable.
Note: do not eat canned vegetables (unless low in salt).

Eau de vie★/*Eau-de-vie*: alcohol beverage made thanks to a distillation process.
Note: do not drink alcoholic beverage, however no problem if it's cooked.

Edam cheese/*Edam*: semi-hard cheese with raw cow's milk. Dairy product.

Edible cortinarius★★★/*Cortinaire comestible*: wild mushroom. Green vegetable.

Edible flower★★★/*Fleur comestible*: flower used as a decoration for a dish and perfectly edible.

Edible mushroom (wild or grown) ★★★/*Champignon comestible (sauvage ou cultivé)*: no-chlorophyll cryptogam. Only a few hundreds of them out of more than 50000 are edible. Green vegetable.
Note: do not eat canned vegetables (unless low in salt).

Edible nutsedge★★★/*Souchet comestible*: plant from which we eat the tubers. Green vegetable.

Eel★★★/*Anguille*: fatty freshwater fish.

Eggnog★★/*Lait de poule*: beverage made thanks to the mixing of a chicken egg yolk in a glass of milk.
Note: do not drink it sweetened.

Eggplant★★/*Aubergine*: annual vegetable plant especially grown in Mediterranean regions. Green vegetable.
Note: do not eat canned vegetables (unless low in salt).

Egg white★/*Blanc d'œuf*: edible part of the egg without the egg yolk.

Egg yolk★★★/*Jaune d'œuf*: yellow part of the egg.

Einkorn bulgur★★★/*Boulgour de petit épeautre*: sieved and crushed einkorn steamed or cooked in water. Carbohydrate.

Einkorn wheat flake★★★/*Flocon de petit-épeautre*: small portion of dehydrated einkorn wheat. Carbohydrate.

Einkorn wheat pasta★★★/*Pâte alimentaire de petit épeautre*: mix to be cooked made of refined einkorn wheat flour. Carbohydrate.

Emmental cheese★★/*Emmental*: hard cow's milk cheese. Dairy product.
Note: consume it in moderation, no more than 1 oz per day of autorized cheese.

Emperor fish★★★/*Capitaine*: saltwater fish with white flesh.

Endive★★/*Endive*: excessive bud which we eat in salad or as a vegetable. Green vegetable.
Note: do not eat canned vegetables (unless low in salt).

Energy drink/*Boisson énergisante*: fizzy or still drink made of taurine and caffeine.

English sauce★★/*Sauce anglaise*: white sauce with chicken stock, Madeira wine and tomato purée.
Note: many commercially prepared foods are high in salt: prepare it yourself without salt and with authorized foods.

Epoisses de Bourgogne/*Epoisses*: soft cow's milk cheese with washed rind. Dairy product.

Escarole★★★/*Scarole*: curly endive with large leaves eaten in salad. Green vegetable.

Espresso★★★/*Expresso*: express coffee rich in caffeine.
Note: do not drink it sweetened.

Eurasian minnow★★★/*Vairon*: small freshwater fish with white flesh.

European barracuda★★★/*Spet*: saltwater fish with white flesh.

European sprat★★★/*Sprat*: fatty saltwater fish.

Exotic fruit★★/*Fruit exotique*: fruit coming from far away foreign countries.
Note: consume it immediately after the meal.

Eye of round★★/*Noix de bœuf*: piece of beef to roast. Red meat.

F

Fajita★★/*Fajita*: corn tortilla. Carbohydrate. Gluten-free.
Note: many commercially prepared foods are high in salt: prepare it yourself without salt and with authorized foods.

Falafel★★/*Falafel*: small fava bean and chickpea doughnut-shaped patty. Carbohydrate. Gluten-free.
Note: many commercially prepared foods are high in salt: prepare it yourself without salt and with authorized foods.

Farmhouse bread/*Pain de campagne*: bread with a thick crust made of leaven and wheat flour milled on a millstone. Carbohydrate.

Fast★★★/*Jeûne*: deprivation of food for a more or less long period of time.

Fatback★★★/*Lard*: adipose piece of the pork.

Fatty fish★★★/*Poisson gras*: fish with brown flesh, rich in omega 3 and in polyunsaturated fats: mackerel, sardine, tuna, herring, trout, char, salmon, anchovy, eel, conger, etc.
Note: do not consume salted and/or smoked fish. A few fatty fish are ★★. Cook it without fat and salt: en papillote, in water, grill, roast...

Fatty fish fillet★★★/*Filet de poisson gras*: slice of fatty fish in general without fishbone.
Note: do not consume salted and/or smoked fish. A few fatty fish fillet are ★★. Cook it without fat and salt: en papillote, in water, grill, roast...

Fatty slice★★★/*Tranche grasse*: piece of beef to grill. Red meat.

Fava bean★★★/*Fève*: seed from a vegetable annual plant. Carbohydrate.

Fennel★★/*Fenouil*: vegetable and aromatic plant from which we eat the plump leafstalk base. Green vegetable.

Fennel seed★★★/*Graine de fenouil*: fennel seed eaten crushed or germinated.

Fenugreek seed★★★/*Graine de fenugrec*: fenugreek seed eaten crushed or germinated.

15% fat ground beef steak★★★/*Steak haché de bœuf à 15% de matières grasses*: ground beef meat containing 15% of fat. To grill.

15% fat lightly salted butter/*Beurre demi-sel à 15% de matières grasses*: lightly salted butter which fat quantity has been reduced from more than three fourths compared to traditional butter.

15% fat lightly unsalted butter★★★/*Beurre doux à 15% de matières grasses*: unsalted butter which fat quantity has been reduced from more than three fourths compared to traditional butter.

Fig jelly/*Pâte de figue*: cf. "Dried fig".

Fillet (beef meat)★★/*Filet (viande de bœuf)*: tender and plump piece of beef. Red meat.

Fillet (lamb meat)★★/*Filet (viande d'agneau)*: tender and plump piece of lamb. Red meat.

Fillet of duck breast★★★/*Magret*: fillet of duck flesh. Red meat.

Fillet (pork meat)★★★/*Filet (viande de porc)*: tender and plump piece of pork.

Fillet (veal meat)★★★/*Filet (viande de veau)*: tender and plump piece of veal.

Financier★★/*Financière*: side dish or sauce made of mushrooms, truffles, sweetbread, etc.
Note: many commercially prepared foods are high in salt: prepare it yourself without salt and with authorized foods.

Findi pasta★★★/*Pâte alimentaire de fonio*: mix to be cooked made of refined findi flour. Carbohydrate. Gluten-free.

Fish pâté en croûte/*Pâté de poisson en croûte*: dish made of ground fish wrapped in puff pastry.

Fish stock★★/*Fumet de poisson*: very reduced stock made of fish.
Note: many commercially prepared foods are high in salt: prepare it yourself without salt and with authorized foods.

Fish terrine/*Pain de poisson*: dish made of potatoes, fish, butter and eggs and served cold with a mayonnaise.

5% fat ground beef steak★★/*Steak haché de bœuf à 5% de matières grasses*: ground beef meat containing 5% of fat. To grill.

5% fat lightly salted butter/*Beurre demi-sel à 5% de matières grasses*: lightly salted butter which fat quantity is very low compared to traditional butter.

5% fat lightly unsalted butter★★★/*Beurre doux à 5% de matières grasses*: unsalted butter which fat quantity is very low compared to traditional butter.

Fizzy water★/*Eau gazeuse*: natural water enriched or naturally rich in carbon dioxide.
Note: almost fizzy waters are too salty.

73

Flageolet★★★/*Flageolet*: seed from a vegetable legume. Carbohydrate.

Flan (mixture)★★/*Flan (appareil à)*: mixture made of eggs, milk, crème fraîche, with or without flour, salted or sweet, to which ingredients (green vegetables, fish, meat, etc.) are added or not.
Note: many commercially prepared foods are high in salt: prepare it yourself without salt and with authorized foods.

Flank (beef)★★/*Flanchet (de bœuf)*: beef meat. Red meat.

Flank steak★★/*Bavette*: tender piece of beef. Red meat.

Flank (veal)★★★/*Flanchet (de veau)*: veal meat.

Flavored yogurt/*Yaourt aromatisé*: goat, sheep or cow's milk fermented thanks to lactic acid bacteria before being sweetened and flavored. Dairy product.

Flax flour★★★/*Farine de lin*: powder made of flax milling. Carbohydrate. Gluten-free.

Flax pasta★★★/*Pâte alimentaire de lin*: mix to be cooked made of flax flour. Carbohydrate. Gluten-free.

Flaxseed★★★/*Graine de lin*: flax seed eaten crushed.

Floating island/*Ile flottante*: caramelized beaten egg white put on custard with grilled almonds.

Flounder★★★/*Flet*: flat saltwater fish with white flesh.

Foie gras/Foie gras: liver which is the result of goose or duck force-feeding. Cooked meat.

Foil or baking parchment parcel★★★/*Papillote*: aluminium sheet used to wrap some foods, usually fresh fish, to steam them or to bake them in the oven without adding any fat and salt.

Fondue★/*Fondue*: dish made of Emmental cheese and gruyère strips melted in white wine.
Note: consume it in moderation, no more than 1 oz per day of autorized cheese.

Fonio flour★★★/*Farine de fonio*: powder made of not whole-grain folio milling. Carbohydrate. Gluten-free.

Fontainebleau cheese/*Fontainebleau*: cow's milk fromage frais. Dairy product.

Fontina/*Fontine*: raw cow's milk semi-hard cheese. Dairy product.

41% fat lightly salted butter/*Beurre demi-sel à 41% de matières grasses*: lightly salted butter which fat quantity is half the quantity of traditional butter.

41% fat lightly unsalted butter★★★/*Beurre doux à 41% de matières grasses*: unsalted butter which fat quantity is half the quantity of traditional butter.

Fourme/*Fourme*: cow's milk cheese. Dairy product.

Foutou★★★/*Foutou*: yam flour cooked in water and served under the shape of a ball. Gluten-free.

Frangipane cream★★/*Crème frangipane*: custard with almond powder. Dairy product.
Note: many commercially prepared foods are high in sugar, so prepare it yourself without sugar and with authorized foods.

French fries★★★/*Frites*: fried potatoes. Carbohydrate. Gluten-free.
Note: do not salt!

French toast/*Pain perdu*: dessert made of stale bread or brioche soaked in milk and in eggs, sweetened and fried. Carbohydrate.

Fresh apple★★★/*Pomme fraîche*: edible fruit from the apple tree.

Fresh apricot★★/*Abricot frais*: fresh fruit from the apricot tree.
Note: consume it immediately after the meal.

Fresh aronia★★/*Aronia fraîche*: little red or black berry. Red fruit.
Note: consume it immediately after the meal.

Fresh azerole★★/*Azerole fraîche*: small red fruit looking like a cherry, very rich in vitamin C.
Note: consume it immediately after the meal.

Fresh blackberry★★/*Mûre fraîche*: edible fruit from the blackberry bush.
Note: consume it immediately after the meal.

Fresh blackcurrant★★/*Cassis frais*: fruit, small black berry.
Note: consume it immediately after the meal.

Fresh button mangosteen★★/*Mangoustan frais*: fruit from the mangosteen. Exotic fruit.
Note: consume it immediately after the meal.

Fresh carambola★★/*Carambole fraîche*: fruit with juicy and acid flesh. Exotic fruit.
Note: consume it immediately after the meal.

Fresh cherimoya★★/*Anone fraîche*: edible tropical fruit. Exotic fruit.
Note: consume it immediately after the meal.

Fresh cherry★★/*Cerise fraîche*: fruit from the cherry tree.
Note: consume it immediately after the meal.

Fresh chili pepper★★★/*Piment frais*: vegetable plant from which we eat the fruit which is more or less spicy. Green vegetable.

Fresh clementine★★/*Clémentine fraîche*: fruit from the clementine tree.
Note: consume it immediately after the meal.

Fresh cocoplum★★/*Icaque fraîche*: edible fruit from the chrysobalanus icaco. Exotic fruit.
Note: consume it immediately after the meal.

Fresh cranberry★★/*Canneberge fraîche*: red berry looking like a vaccinium. Red fruit.
Note: consume it immediately after the meal.

Fresh date★★/*Datte fraîche*: fruit from the date palm. Exotic fruit.
Note: consume it immediately after the meal.

Fresh fig★★/*Figue fraîche*: fresh fruit from the fig tree.
Note: consume it immediately after the meal.

Fresh fruit/*Fruit frais*: apple, pear, banana, etc. See each of them depending on their own name.

Fresh fruit salad★★/*Salade de fruits frais*: mix of various fresh fruits without adding anything.
Note: consume it immediately after the meal.

Fresh goji berry★★/*Baie de goji fraîche*: small red berry from a Chinese bush.
Note: consume it immediately after the meal.

Fresh grape★★/*Raisin frais*: fruit from the vine.
Note: consume it immediately after the meal.

Fresh grapefruit★★/*Pamplemousse frais*: edible fruit from the grapefruit tree.
Note: consume it immediately after the meal.

Fresh green vegetable preserved after being cooked - Fresh mackerel

Fresh green vegetable preserved after being cooked/*Légume vert frais cuisiné en conserve*: fresh green vegetable treated in various industrial ways before being put in cans.

Fresh green vegetable preserved without being cooked/*Légume vert frais en conserve non cuisiné*: fresh green vegetable, blanched before being preserved in brine and put in cans.

Fresh guava★★/*Goyave fraîche*: fruit from the common guava. Exotic fruit.
Note: consume it immediately after the meal.

Fresh jujube★★/*Jujube fraîche*: fruit from the ziziphus. Exotic fruit.
Note: consume it immediately after the meal.

Fresh kaki★★/*Kaki frais*: fruit from the date plum tree.
Note: consume it immediately after the meal.

Fresh kiwi★★/*Kiwi frais*: fruit from the actinidia.
Note: consume it immediately after the meal.

Fresh kumquat★★/*Kumquat frais*: fruit from the kumquat, yellow citrus fruit.
Note: consume it immediately after the meal.

Fresh lemon★★★/*Citron frais*: fruit from the lemon tree.

Fresh longan★★/*Longane fraîche*: fruit from the longan tree. Exotic fruit.
Note: consume it immediately after the meal.

Fresh lychee★★/*Litchi frais*: fruit from the lychee. Exotic fruit.
Note: consume it immediately after the meal.

Fresh mackerel★★/*Maquereau frais*: fatty saltwater fish freshly caught.

Fresh malay rose apple★★/***Jambose fraîche***: fruit from the syzygium malaccense. Exotic fruit.
Note: consume it immediately after the meal.

Fresh mandarin★★/***Mandarine fraîche***: fruit from the mandarin tree.
Note: consume it immediately after the meal.

Fresh mango★★/***Mangue fraîche***: fruit from the mango tree. Exotic fruit.
Note: consume it immediately after the meal.

Fresh medlar★★/***Nèfle fraîche***: fruit from the medlar tree eaten overripe.
Note: consume it immediately after the meal.

Fresh melon★★/***Melon frais***: fruit from the cucurbits family.
Note: consume it immediately after the meal.

Fresh mirabelle plum★★/***Mirabelle fraîche***: small yellow plum.
Note: consume it immediately after the meal.

Fresh mombins★★/***Mombin frais***: fruit from spondias. Exotic fruit.
Note: consume it immediately after the meal.

Fresh mulberries★★/***Mulberries fraîche***: small berry very similar to the blackberry but longer.
Note: consume it immediately after the meal.

Fresh myrciaria★★/***Camu-camu fraîche***: red orangey fruit looking like a plum and rich in vitamin C. Exotic fruit.
Note: consume it immediately after the meal.

Fresh nectarine★★/***Brugnon frais***: fruit from the nectarine tree.
Note: consume it immediately after the meal.

Fresh orange★★/*Orange fraîche*: fruit from the orange tree.
Note: consume it immediately after the meal.

Fresh papaya★★/*Papaye fraîche*: fruit from the papaya tree. Exotic fruit.
Note: consume it immediately after the meal.

Fresh passion fruit★★/*Fruit de la passion frais*: fruit from some varieties of passion vine. Exotic fruit.
Note: consume it immediately after the meal.

Fresh peach★★/*Pêche fraîche*: edible fruit from the peach tree.
Note: consume it immediately after the meal.

Fresh pear★★/*Poire fraîche*: fruit from the pear tree.
Note: consume it immediately after the meal.

Fresh physalis★★/*Physalis fraîche*: small round fruit. Exotic fruit.
Note: consume it immediately after the meal.

Fresh pineapple★★/*Ananas frais*: big tropical fruit with sugary and tasty flesh. Exotic fruit.
Note: consume it immediately after the meal.

Fresh pitaya★★/*Pitaya fraîche*: exotic fruit also called dragon fruit.
Note: consume it immediately after the meal.

Fresh plum★★/*Prune fraîche*: fruit from the plum tree.
Note: consume it immediately after the meal.

Fresh pomegranate★★/*Grenade fraîche*: fruit from the pomegranate tree. Exotic fruit.
Note: consume it immediately after the meal.

Fresh quince★★/*Coing frais*: yellow fruit from the quince tree.
Note: consume it immediately after the meal.

Fresh rambutan★★/*Ramboutan frais*: fruit from the rambutan. Exotic fruit.
Note: consume it immediately after the meal.

Fresh raspberry★★/*Framboise fraîche*: fresh fruit from the raspberry bush.
Note: consume it immediately after the meal.

Fresh redcurrant★★/*Groseille fraîche*: edible fruit from the currant bush.
Note: consume it immediately after the meal.

Fresh salak★★/*Salacca frais*: fruit from a palm family, exotic fruit.
Note: consume it immediately after the meal.

Fresh salmon★★★/*Saumon frais*: fatty fish found in freshwater.

Fresh sapodilla fruit★★/*Sapotille fraîche*: fruit from the sapodilla. Exotic fruit.
Note: consume it immediately after the meal.

Fresh sardine★/*Sardine fraîche*: fatty saltwater fish freshly caught.

Fresh sloe★★/*Prunelle fraîche*: fruit from the sloe tree.
Note: consume it immediately after the meal.

Fresh sorb★★/*Sorbe fraîche*: fruit from the sorb tree.
Note: consume it immediately after the meal.

Fresh strawberry★★★/*Fraise fraîche*: plump fruit from the strawberry plant.

Fresh tamarind fruit★★/*Tamarin frais*: fruit from the tamarind. Laxative exotic fruit.
Note: consume it immediately after the meal.

Fresh tuna★★★/*Thon frais*: fatty saltwater fish freshly caught.

Freshwater fish★★★/*Poisson de rivière*: every fatty and lean fish found in rivers.
Note: do not consume salted and/or smoked fish. A few freshwater fish are ★★. Cook it without fat and salt: en papillote, in water, grill, roast...

Fresh watermelon★★★/*Pastèque fraîche*: big fruit with very juicy red flesh.

Fried egg★★★/*Œuf au plat*: lightly cooked egg, not scrambled, in an oiled frying pan.

Fried food/*Friture*: cf. "Fry".

Frikandel★★/*Fricadelle*: small ball of ground meat.
Note: many commercially prepared foods are high in salt: prepare it yourself without salt and with authorized foods.

Fritter★★/*Beignet*: fried dish consisting of a piece of meat, fruit, vegetable, etc. wrapped in a thick batter or breading.
Note: many commercially prepared foods are high in salt and/or in sugar so prepare it yourself without salt and sugar and with authorized foods.

Frog's leg★★★/*Cuisse de grenouille*: edible frog's leg.

Fromage à la pie/*Fromage à la pie*: cow's milk fromage frais with herbs. Dairy product.

Fructose★/*Fructose*: component of the sugar used as sweetener.

Fruit bar/*Barre de fruits*: very sugary bar made of various dried or fresh fruits.

Fruit compote★★/*Compote de fruit*: mix of fresh or dried fruits cooked with a little bit of water and added sugar.
Note: consume it immediately after the meal.

Fruit compote with no added sugar★★★/*Compote de fruit sans sucre ajouté*: mix of fresh or dried fruits cooked without added sugar.
Note: consume it immediately after the meal.

Fruit in light syrup★/*Fruit au sirop léger*: fruit poached in a syrup made of water and a small quantity of sugar.
Note: consume it immediately after the meal.

Fruit in light syrup cocktail★/*Cocktail de fruit au sirop léger*: mix of various fruits cut in dices and poached before being preserved in more or less sugary water.
Note: consume it immediately after the meal.

Fruit in syrup/*Fruit au sirop*: poached fruit preserved in a syrup made of water and sugar.

Fruit in syrup cocktail/*Cocktail de fruit au sirop*: mix of various fruits cut in dices and poached before being preserved in very sugary water.

Fruit jelly(1) /*Gelée de fruit*: fruit juice cooked with sugar and which hardens when cooling.

Fruit jelly(2)/*Pâte de fruit*: confection made of fruit purée and sugar.

Fruit juice with pulp/*Jus de fruit avec pulpe*: 100% pure juice fruit juice with the pulp.

Fruit Melba/*Fruit Melba*: fruit poached in syrup before being served on a layer of vanilla ice cream and coated with whipped cream.

Fruit nectar/*Nectar de fruits*: beverage made of fruit purée with water and sugar.

Fruit pectin/*Pectine de fruit*: very sugary substance extracted from fruits used to set jams and sugar-coat pastries.

Fruit salad in light syrup★/*Salade de fruits au sirop léger*: mix of various fresh fruits preserved in their low-sugar poaching syrup.

Fruit salad in syrup/*Salade de fruits au sirop*: mix of various poached fruits preserved in their poaching syrup.

Fruit specialty/*Spécialité de fruit*: fruit cooked with fructose and fruit pectin.

Fruit yogurt/*Yaourt aux fruits*: cow's milk, goat milk or sheep milk fermented thanks to lactic acid bacteria and in which fruits have been added. Dairy product.

Fucus vesiculosus/*Fucus vésiculeux*: edible seaweed.

Fufu★★/*Foufou*: cassava flour cooked in water and served under the shape of a ball. Gluten-free.
Note: many commercially prepared foods are high in salt: prepare it yourself without salt and with authorized foods.

G

Galantine/*Galantine*: cooked meat made of lean meat and stuffing covered with jelly.

Galette bretonne/*Galette bretonne*: plain cookie rich in sugar and butter.

Galloway cheese: raw or pasteurised cow's milk cheese. Dairy product.

Game★★★/*Gibier*: all wild animals hunted for their meat.

Ganache★★/*Crème ganache*: chocolate custard with butter and crème fraîche.
Note: many commercially prepared foods are high in sugar, so prepare it yourself without sugar and with authorized foods.

Gaperon/*Gaperon*: soft raw cow's milk cheese flavored with garlic. Dairy product.

Garden orache: cf. "Atriplex hortensis".

Garden sage★★★/*Thé d'Europe*: infusion of heath speedwell leaves.
Note: do not drink it sweetened.

Garfish★★★/*Orphie*: long, thin and fatty saltwater fish.

Garlic★★★/*Ail*: vegetable bulb-plant which cloves are used when cooking. Green vegetable.

Garlic pulp/Pulpe d'ail: cf. "Garlic".

Garlic salt/*Sel d'ail*: mix of table salt and dehydrated garlic in powder.

Garlic sausage/*Saucisson à l'ail*: big sausage eaten cooked. Cooked meat.

Garlic semolina★★★/*Ail semoule*: dehydrated and crushed garlic.

Gazpacho - Germinated mung bean seed

Gazpacho★★/*Gaspacho*: soup made of raw vegetables macerated in cold water and served very fresh. Green vegetable.
Note: many commercially prepared foods are high in salt: prepare it yourself without salt and with authorized foods.

Gelatin★★★/*Gélatine*: collagen sheet which dissolves in hot water to make jellies.

Genoise★★/*Génoise*: light cookie dough used as the base of numerous cakes.
Note: many commercially prepared foods are high in salt and/or in sugar so prepare it yourself without salt and sugar and with authorized foods.

Germinated adzuki bean seed★★★/*Graine de haricot azuki germée*: adzuki bean seed eaten germinated.

Germinated barley seed★★★/*Graine d'orge germée*: barley seed eaten germinated.

Germinated buckwheat seed★★★/*Graine de sarrasin germée*: buckwheat seed eaten germinated.

Germinated chickpea seed★★★/*Graine de pois chiche germée*: chickpea seed eaten germinated.

Germinated corn grain★★★/*Graine de maïs germée*: corn grain eaten germinated.

Germinated lentil seed★★★/*Graine de lentille germée*: lentil seed eaten germinated.

Germinated millet seed★★★/*Graine de millet germée*: millet seed eaten germinated.

Germinated mung bean seed★★★/*Graine de haricot mungo germée*: muni bean seed eaten germinated.

Germinated oats seed★★★/*Graine d'avoine germée*: oats seed eaten germinated.

Germinated pea seed★★/*Graine de petit pois germée*: pea seed eaten germinated.

Germinated rice seed★★★/*Graine de riz germée*: rice seed eaten germinated.

Germinated rye seed★★★/*Graine de seigle germée*: rye seed eaten germinated.

Germinated spelt seed★★★/*Graine d'épeautre germée*: spelt seed eaten germinated.

Germinated wheat seed★★★/*Graine de blé germée*: wheat seed eaten germinated.

Giblets★/**Abats de volaille**: edible offal of a fowl, typically including the heart, gizzard, liver, and other organs.

Gigot★★/*Gigot*: lamb, sheep or deer posterior. Red meat.

Gin/*Gin*: grain eau de vie flavored with juniper berries.

Ginger★★★/*Gingembre*: aromatic rhizome used as a condiment. Green vegetable.

Gingerbread/*Pain d'épice*: cake made of rye flour with sugar, honey and seasoning. Carbohydrate.

Gizzard★★/*Gésier*: poultry stomach. Offal.

Glucose/*Glucose*: carbohydrate, quick sugar.

Gluten★★★/*Gluten*: protein part of the following cereals: wheat, rye, barley and oats.

Gluten-free bagel/*Bagel sans gluten*: small white bread shaped into a ring with very firm gluten-free crumb. Carbohydrate.

Gluten-free beer★/*Bière sans gluten*: drink from the alcoholic fermentation of mainly barley and from which the gluten is extracted.
Note: do not drink alcoholic beverage, however no problem if it's cooked.

Gluten-free bread/*Pain sans gluten*: bread made of gluten-free flour. Carbohydrate.

Gluten-free breadcrumbs/*Chapelure sans gluten*: gluten-free white bread toasted in the oven before being crushed into crumbs. Carbohydrate.

Gluten-free breakfast sugary extruded cereal/*Céréale extrudée sucrée pour petit-déjeuner sans gluten*: gluten-free swelled cereal coated in sugar, honey, chocolat, etc. Carbohydrate.

Gluten-free bun/*Bun sans gluten*: small round and puffy gluten-free bread. Carbohydrate.

Gluten-free cake(1)/*Cake sans gluten*: cake made of gluten-free egg batter with yeast, candied fruits and raisins soaked in rum.

Gluten-free cake(2)/*Gâteau sans gluten*: pastry made of a gluten-free batter used alone or with a cream, fruits...

Gluten-free cannellonis/*Cannelloni sans gluten*: gluten-free pasta rolled in the shape of a cylinder and stuffed with stuffing. Carbohydrate.

Gluten-free cookie/*Biscuit sans gluten*: cookie that does not contain gluten. Carbohydrate.

Gluten-free crepe★★/*Crêpe sans gluten*: crepe made of gluten-free flour.
Note: many commercially prepared foods are high in salt and/or in sugar so prepare it yourself without salt and sugar and with authorized foods.

Gluten-free crispbread/*Biscotte sans gluten*: slice of gluten-free sandwich bread industrially toasted in the oven. Carbohydrate.

Gluten-free crouton/*Croûton sans gluten*: small piece of fried gluten-free white bread. Carbohydrate.

Gluten-free kringle/*Craquelin sans gluten*: small crispy cookie made of an unleavened and gluten-free batter.

Gluten-free madeleine/*Madeleine sans gluten*: small cake in the shape of a bulging shell made of gluten-free flour.

Gluten-free margarine★★/*Margarine sans gluten*: gluten-free plant-based dietary fats.
Note: only if it's unsalted.

Gluten-free muffin/*Muffin sans gluten*: small plain bread with leaven but without gluten. Carbohydrate.

Gluten-free pancakes★★/*Pancakes sans gluten*: small thick crepe made of gluten-free sieved flour. Carbohydrate.
Note: many commercially prepared foods are high in salt and/or in sugar so prepare it yourself without salt and sugar and with authorized foods.

Gluten-free pie crust★★/*Pâte brisée sans gluten*: crust made of gluten-free flour, butter and eggs. Carbohydrate.
Note: many commercially prepared foods are high in salt: prepare it yourself without salt and with authorized foods.

Gluten-free pizza base
- Gluten-free wholewheat breadcrumbs

Gluten-free pizza base★ ★/*Pâte à pizza sans gluten*: base made of gluten-free flour, water and yeast.
Note: many commercially prepared foods are high in salt: prepare it yourself without salt and with authorized foods.

Gluten-free pretzel/*Bretzel sans gluten*: gluten-free cookie into an 8-shape, sprinkled with salt and cumin.

Gluten-free puff pastry★ ★/*Pâte feuilletée sans gluten*: pastry made of gluten-free flour, butter and eggs. Carbohydrate.
Note: many commercially prepared foods are high in salt: prepare it yourself without salt and with authorized foods.

Gluten-free sweet shortcrust pastry★ ★/*Pâte sablée sans gluten*: pastry made of gluten-free flour, sugar, butter and eggs.
Note: many commercially prepared foods are high in salt and/or in sugar so prepare it yourself without salt and sugar and with authorized foods.

Gluten-free toast/*Toast sans gluten*: slice of gluten-free toasted bread.

Gluten-free whole-grain cannellonis/*Cannelloni complet sans gluten*: whole-grain gluten-free pasta rolled in the shape of a cylinder and stuffed with stuffing. Carbohydrate.

Gluten-free whole-grain muffin/*Muffin complet sans gluten*: small plain whole-grain bread with leaven but without gluten. Carbohydrate.

Gluten-free wholewheat breadcrumbs/*Chapelure complète sans gluten*: gluten-free wholewheat bread toasted in the oven before being crushed into crumbs. Carbohydrate.

Gluten-free wholewheat crepe★★/*Crêpe complète sans gluten*: thin layer of cooked batter made of eggs, milk and gluten-free wholewheat flour. Carbohydrate.
Note: many commercially prepared foods are high in salt and/or in sugar so prepare it yourself without salt and sugar and with authorized foods.

Gluten-free wholewheat crouton/*Croûton complet sans gluten*: small piece of fried gluten-free wholewheat bread. Carbohydrate.

Gluten-free wholewheat pancakes★★/*Pancakes complet sans gluten*: small thick crepes made of gluten-free wholewheat flour. Carbohydrate.
Note: many commercially prepared foods are high in salt and/or in sugar so prepare it yourself without salt and sugar and with authorized foods.

Gluten-free wholewheat toast/*Toast complet sans gluten*: slice of gluten-free wholewheat toasted bread.

Gnocchi★★/*Gnocchi*: ball made of wheat semolina and potatoes. Carbohydrate.
Note: many commercially prepared foods are high in salt: prepare it yourself without salt and with authorized foods.

Goat milk cheese★/*Fromage de chèvre*: cheese made of goat milk. Dairy product.
Note: almost all cheeses are too salty.

Goat milk cottage cheese★★★/*Faisselle au lait de chèvre*: fresh cheese made of goat milk. Dairy product.

Goat milk cream dessert/*Crème dessert au lait de chèvre*: dairy specialty or dessert made of goat milk, sugar and eggs. Dairy product.

Goat milk fromage blanc★★★/*Fromage blanc de chèvre*: fresh cheese made of goat milk, a bit drained and not aged. Dairy product.

Goat's cheese log/*Bûche de chèvre*: goat milk cheese in the shape of a small round and long cylinder. Dairy product.

Gomashio/*Gomasio*: sesame and sea salt condiment.

Good-king-Henry: cf. "Blitum bonus-henricus".

Goose★★★/*Oie*: massive palmiped bird. Poultry.

Goose fat★★★/*Graisse d'oie*: goose fat used to make confits.

Goose rillettes/*Rillettes d'oie*: cooked meat made of goose meat cooked in its fat.

Gorgonzola/*Gorgonzola*: cow's milk cheese with parsley in it. Dairy product.

Gouda/*Gouda*: pressed and raw cow's milk cheese. Dairy product.

Gougère/*Gougère*: salted choux pastry with gruyère baked in the oven.

Goulash★★/*Goulache*: stew made of simmered meat, onions, tomatoes and paprika.
Note: many commercially prepared foods are high in salt: prepare it yourself without salt and with authorized foods.

Grapefruit in light syrup★/*Pamplemousse au sirop léger*: poached grapefruit preserved in more or less sugary water.

Grapefruit in syrup/*Pamplemousse au sirop*: poached grapefruit preserved in very sugary water.

Grapefruit juice/*Jus de pamplemousse*: juice made of the pressing of grapefruits.

Grape juice/*Jus de raisin*: juice made of the pressing of grapes.

Grape seed oil★★★/*Huile de pépin de raisin*: fatty substance made of grape seeds.

Grated coconut/*Noix de coco râpée*: cf. "Coconut". Exotic fruit.

Gratin/*Gratin*: dish covered with breadcrumbs or cheese baked in the oven.

Grayling★★★/*Ombre*: fatty freshwater fish.

Grecque (à la)★★/*Grecque (à la)*: cooked in an olive oil and seasoning marinade, eaten cold.
Note: many commercially prepared foods are high in salt: prepare it yourself without salt and with authorized foods.

Greek yogurt/*Yaourt à la grecque*: cf. "Yogurt".
Green bean★★/*Haricot vert*: green or violet bean, sometimes green with black stripes or brown, chocolate... eaten young. Green vegetable.
Note: do not eat canned vegetables (unless low in salt).

Green laver★★★/*Ao-nori*: edible green seaweeds.
Note: do not eat canned vegetables (unless low in salt).

Green tea★★★/*Thé vert*: infusion of tea bush leaves roasted after being picked.
Note: do not drink it sweetened.

Green vegetable cream soup/*Velouté de légumes verts*: cf. "Green vegetable soup".

Green vegetable/*Légume vert*: vegetable plant from which, depending on the variety, we eat the leaves, the chards, the stems, the roots or the fruits. See each green vegetable separately.

Green vegetable soup★★/*Potage de légumes verts*: mixed vegetable stock.
Note: many commercially prepared foods are high in salt: prepare it yourself without salt and with authorized foods.

Green vegetable soup in carton/*Potage de légumes verts en brique*: industrial soup ready to be drunk.

Grenadine/*Grenadine*: syrup flavored with red berry juice and vanilla.

Grenadine juice/*Jus de grenade*: juice made of the pressing of pomegranates. Exotic fruit.

Grilled buckwheat★★★/*Sarrasin grillé*: grilled buckwheat seed ready to be eaten.

Grilled food★★★/*Grillade*: slice of meat or grilled fish.

Grilletine/*Grilletine*: slice of brioche toasted in the oven. Carbohydrate.

Grissino/*Gressin*: small white bread made with an egg batter. Carbohydrate.

Ground beef steak with vegetable protein★★★/*Steak haché de bœuf avec protéines végétales*: ground beef steak containing 80% of ground beef meat and 20% of vegetable proteins.

Ground (food)★★★/*Haché (aliment)*: food that is ground before being eaten.

Ground ham steak/*Steak haché de jambon*: ground pork meat.

Ground meat★★/*Hachis*: dish made of ground meat, fish, green vegetables.
Note: many commercially prepared foods are high in salt: prepare it yourself without salt and with authorized foods.

Groundnut★★★/*Arachide*: envelope of the peanut.
Note: only if it's unsalted.

Groundnut butter/*Beurre d'arachide*: cf. "Peanut".

Ground veal steak★★★/*Steak haché de veau*: ground veal meat.

Grouper★★★/*Mérou*: saltwater fish with white flesh found in hot waters.

Gruel★★★/*Gruau*: hard wheat semolina. Carbohydrate.

Gruel flour★★★/*Farine de gruau*: sieved and very thin wheat of high quality flour. Carbohydrate.

Gruyère★★/*Gruyère*: hard cow's milk with washed rind. Dairy product.
Note: consume it in moderation, no more than 1 oz per day of autorized cheese.

Guacamole★★/*Guacamole*: dish made of avocados, tomatoes, onions, crème fraîche and spices.
Note: many commercially prepared foods are high in salt: prepare it yourself without salt and with authorized foods.

Guar gum★★★/*Gomme de guar*: vegetable thickening substance.

Guava in light syrup★/*Goyave au sirop léger*: poached guava preserved in more or less sugary water. Exotic fruit.

Guava in syrup/*Goyave au sirop*: poached guava preserved in very sugary water. Exotic fruit.

Guava jelly/*Pâte de goyave*: sugary guava marmalade.

Guava juice/Jus de goyave: juice made of the pressing of guavas. Exotic fruit.

Gudgeon★★★/*Goujon*: small freshwater fish with white flesh.

Guinea fowl★★★/*Pintade*: bird a little bit smaller than chicken.

Gurnard★★★/*Grondin*: saltwater fish with white flesh.

ℋ

Haddock★★★/*Eglefin*: saltwater fish with white flesh.

Halbi/*Halbi*: beverage made of a mix of fermented apples and pears.

Halibut★★★/*Flétan*: big saltwater fish with white flesh.

Halibut liver oil★★★/*Huile de foie de flétan*: fatty substance made of halibut liver.

Halva/*Halva*: confection made of flour, sesame oil, dried fruits and honey.

Ham/*Jambon blanc*: cooked and boneless pork ham. Cooked meat.

Ham allumette/*Allumette de jambon*: matchstick-sized cut of ham.

Ham and cheese escalope/*Cordon bleu de jambon*: pork escalope wrapped around ham and cheese.

Hamburger(1)★★/*Hamburger(1)*: ground steak in a small round bun. Red meat.

Hamburger(2)★★/*Hamburger(2)*: ground steak with a fried egg. Red meat.

Ham ravioli/*Ravioli au jambon*: small square of pasta stuffed with pork meat, ground herbs, etc. before being poached. Carbohydrate.

Hang★★★/*Faisander*: to give a strong fumet to game letting it start rotting.

Hanger steak★★/*Onglet*: piece of beef from which we cut tasty beefsteaks. Red meat.

Hard-boiled egg★★★/*Œuf dur*: egg cooked in a lot of water.

Hare★★★/*Lièvre*: kind of wild rabbit. Game.

Harissa★/*Harissa*: condiment made of chili pepper and oil.

Haunch★★/*Cuissot*: wild boar's leg, venison's leg or deer's leg. Red meat. Game.

Hazelnut★★★/*Noisette*: nut from the hazel.

Hazelnut cream★★★/*Crème de noisette*: more or less liquid cream made of hazelnut milk, substitute to crème fraîche.

Hazelnut milk★★/*Lait de noisette*: plant milk from hazelnuts. Lactose-free.
Note: do not consume it sweetened.

Hazelnut milk cream dessert/*Crème dessert au lait de noisette*: vegetable dessert made of hazelnut milk, sugar and eggs. Dairy product.

Hazelnut milk yogurt★★/*Yaourt au lait de noisette*: hazelnut milk fermented thanks to lactic acid bacteria, sweetened or not. Dairy product. Lactose-free.
Note: do not consume it sweetened.

Hazelnut oil★★★/*Huile de noisette*: fatty substance made of hazelnut.

Hazelnut purée★★★/*Purée de noisette*: mashed hazelnuts to spread.

Hazelnut spread/*Pâte à tartiner de noisette*: very sugary and fat mix of crushed hazelnuts.

Head cheese/*Fromage de tête*: cooked meat. Pâté made of pork head pieces with jelly.

Headcheese/*Museau*: cooked meat dish made of pork or beef chin and nose.

Heart★★★/*Cœur*: butcher's meat. Offal.

Heavy crème fraîche★★★/*Crème fraîche entière*: fats from unsterilized milk (30%) with which the butter is made. Made of raw milk. Dairy product.

Heifer lamb★★/*Rognon de génisse*: kidney of the heifer. Offal.

Heifer liver★★★/*Foie de génisse*: offal.

Helianthus strumosus★★★/*Hélianti*: vegetable plant from which we eat the rhizome. Green vegetable.

Helvella★★★/*Helvelle*: edible wild mushroom. Green vegetable.

Hemp cream★★★/*Crème de chanvre*: more or less liquid cream made of hemp milk, substitute to crème fraîche.

Hemp milk★★/*Lait de chanvre*: plant milk from hemps. Lactose-free.
Note: do not consume it sweetened.

Hemp milk cream dessert/*Crème dessert au lait de chanvre*: vegetable dessert made of hemp milk, sugar and eggs. Dairy product.

Hemp oil★★★/*Huile de chanvre*: fatty substance made of hemp.

Hemp seed★★★/*Graine de chanvre*: hemp seed eaten crushed or germinated.

Hen★★★/*Poule*: female rooster. Needs to be cooked for a long time, in sauce or boiled. Poultry.

Herbal tea★★★/*Infusion*: liquid in which a plant is put to infuse.
Note: do not drink it sweetened.

Herbs★★★/*Herbes (fines)*: aromatic and edible plants used as condiments: parsley, dill, chive, etc.

Herring★/*Hareng*: fatty saltwater fish.

Hijiki/*Hijiki*: edible black seaweed.

Himanthalia elongata/*Haricot de mer*: edible seaweed.

Hog/*Cochon*: cf. "Pork (meat)".

Hollandaise sauce★★/*Sauce hollandaise*: sauce made of egg yolks and butter.
Note: many commercially prepared foods are high in salt: prepare it yourself without salt and with authorized foods.

Honey/*Miel*: very sugary substance produced by bees.

Hoop cheese: pasteurised cow's milk cheese. Dairy product.

Horse (meat)★★★/*Cheval (viande de...)*: red meat, butcher meat.

Horseradish★★★/*Raifort*: vegetable plant grown for its plump and pepper flavored root. Green vegetable.

Horseradish seed/*Graine de raifort*: horseradish seed eaten crushed or germinated.

Horse spider steak★★★/*Araignée de cheval*: piece of very tender meat from the horse's pelvis muscles. Red meat.

Host★★★/*Hostie*: eucharistic bread made of leaven-free flour. Carbohydrate.
Note: just one, no more!

Hot dog/*Hot dog*: small hot bread with a sausage and mustard.

Hot pot★★/*Fondue chinoise*: dish made of small dices of beef dipped in meat or poultry stock.
Note: many commercially prepared foods are high in salt: prepare it yourself without salt and with authorized foods.

Humboldt fog cheese: pasteurised goat's milk cheese. Dairy product.

Hummus★★/*Houmous*: mix of tahini and mashed split peas. Carbohydrate.
Note: many commercially prepared foods are high in salt: prepare it yourself without salt and with authorized foods.

I

Ice cream(1) /*Crème glacée*: dessert made of cream, milk, sugar and flavors with sometimes egg yolks.

Ice cream(2) /*Glace*: frozen cream made of milk, sugar, eggs fruit-flavored or fruits with fruits.

Iced chocolate with whipped cream/*Liégeois (chocolat)*: chocolate ice cream coated with whipped cream.

Iced tea/*Thé glacé*: infusion of sugary tea drunk fresh.

Industrial ready-cooked dishes/*Plat cuisiné industriel*: various dishes sold vacuum packed, frozen or fresh, industrially made and ready to be eaten.

Industrial sandwich bread/*Pain de mie industriel*: crustless bread made of white flour, industrially produced and sold pre-sliced. Carbohydrate.

Industrial tomato sauce/*Sauce tomate cuisinée*: industrially cooked tomatoes with flavors, meat, additives, etc. found in cans.

Industrial vinaigrette sauce/*Sauce vinaigrette industrielle*: sauce industrially made of vegetable oil and vinegar.

Industrial wholewheat sandwich bread/*Pain de mie complet industriel*: crustless bread made of wholewheat or semi wholewheat flour, industrially produced and sold pre-sliced. Carbohydrate.

Infant formula milk★★★/*Lait pour nourrisson*: food preparation made to replace human breast milk if the mother cannot or do not want to breastfeed her baby.

Irish coffee/*Irish-coffee*: coffee with Irish whiskey and coated with crème fraîche.

Irish moss/*Mousse d'Irlande*: edible red seaweed.

J

Jackfruit★★★/*Jaque*: fruit from the jackfruit tree eaten raw as a vegetable.
Note: do not eat canned vegetables (unless low in salt).

Jam/*Confiture*: mix of fresh fruits and sugar cooked together.

Jam with no sugar★/*Confiture sans sucre*: mix of fruits and sweetener(s) and/or fruit sugar.
Note: consume it immediately after the meal.

John dory★★★/*Saint-pierre*: saltwater fish with white flesh.

Jonchée cheese/*Jonchée*: cow's milk, sheep milk or goat milk cheese in a bulrush basket. Dairy product.

Jujube in light syrup★/*Jujube au sirop léger*: poached jujube preserved in more or less sugary water. Exotic fruit.

Jujube in syrup/*Jujube au sirop*: poached jujube preserved in very sugary water. Exotic fruit.

Jumbo shrimp/*Langoustine*: crustacean the size of a big crawfish.

Junk-food/Fast-food: fast food.

K

Kaki in light syrup★/*Kaki au sirop léger*: poached kaki preserved in more or less sugary water.

Kaki in syrup/*Kaki au sirop*: poached kaki preserved in very sugary water.

Kale★★★/*Chou frisé*: vegetable plant from which we eat all the leaves.
Note: do not eat canned vegetables (unless low in salt).

Kangaroo (meat of...)★★★/*Kangourou (viande de...)*: meat similar to that of beef. Red meat.

Kaoliang liquor/*Kaoliang*: cf. "Sorghum".

Kefir★★★/*Kéfir*: fizzy fermented beverage made of cow's milk, goat milk, sheep milk or she-camel milk. Dairy product.

Ketchup/*Ketchup*: thick spicy sauce made of tomatoes and sugar.

Khorasan wheat flake★★★/*Flocon de kamut*: small portion of dehydrated khorasan wheat. Carbohydrate.

Khorasan wheat flour★★★/*Farine de kamut*: powder made of refined khorasan wheat milling. Carbohydrate.

Khorasan wheat milk★★★/*Lait de kamut*: plant milk from Khorasan wheat. Lactose-free.

Khorasan wheat pasta★★★/*Pâte alimentaire de kamut*: mix to be cooked made of refined khorasan wheat. Carbohydrate.

Kidney bean★★★/*Haricot rouge*: red bean seed eaten fully ripe. Carbohydrate.

Kig ha far★★/*Kig ha far*: pork stew in which a mix of wheat or buckwheat is cooked. Carbohydrate.
Note: many commercially prepared foods are high in salt: prepare it yourself without salt and with authorized foods.

King shrimp/*Gamba*: very big shrimp.

Kipper/*Kipper*: herring which head has been removed before opening the fish and smoking it.

Kir royal/*Kir royal*: champagne with blackcurrant liqueur.

Kir/*Kir*: white wine with blackcurrant liqueur.

Kirsch★/*Kirsch*: cherry eau de vie.
Note: do not drink alcoholic beverage, however no problem if it's cooked.

Kiwi in light syrup★/*Kiwi au sirop léger*: poached kiwi preserved in more or less sugary water.

Kiwi in syrup/*Kiwi au sirop*: poached kiwi preserved in very sugary water.

Kiwi juice/*Jus de kiwi*: juice made of the pressing of kiwis.

Kohlrabi★★★/*Chou-rave*: vegetable plant from which we eat the stem bulge.

Kombu/*Kombu*: edible seaweed.

Kringle/*Craquelin*: small crispy cookie made of an unleavened batter.

Kumis/Koumis: fermented beverage made of cow's milk, mare's milk or she-camel milk. Dairy product.

Kumquat in light syrup★/*Kumquat au sirop léger*: poached kumquat preserved in more or less sugary water.

Kumquat in syrup/*Kumquat au sirop*: poached kumquat preserved in very sugary water.

Kvass/*Kwas*: alcoholic beverage made of fermented barley or rye flour.

L

Lactose-free butter★★/*Beurre sans lactose*: unsalted dietary fats made from the cream of lactose-free cow's milk.
Note: only if it's unsalted.

Lactose-free fromage blanc★★★/*Fromage blanc sans lactose* : fresh cheese made of lactose-free milk, a bit drained and not aged. Dairy product.

Lactose-free margarine★★/*Margarine sans lactose*: lactose-free plant-based dietary fats.
Note: only if it's unsalted.

Lactose-free petit suisse★★★/*Petit-suisse sans lactose*: plain petit suisse made of lactose-free milk.

Lactose-free semi-skimmed milk★★★/*Lait demi-écrémé délactosé*: lactose-free mammal milk which has been semi skimmed.

Lactose-free skimmed milk★★★/*Lait écrémé délactosé*: skimmed mammal milk without lactose.

Lactose-free whole milk★★★/*Lait entier délactosé*: whole mammal milk without lactose.

Lactose-free yogurt★★/*Yaourt sans lactose*: mammal milk yogurt without lactose. Dairy product.
Note: do not consume it sweetened.

Ladyfinger/*Boudoir*: long cookie sprinkled with sugar.

Laguiole cheese/*Laguiole*: raw cow's milk cheese close to Cantal cheese. Dairy product.

Lamb breast★★/*Poitrine d'agneau*: inferior part of the lamb's rib cage to boil or to simmer. Red meat.

Lamb kidney/*Rognon d'agneau*: kidney of the lamb. Offal.

Lamb liver★★★/*Foie d'agneau*: offal.

Lamb (meat)/*Agneau (viande d')*: baby of the sheep. Red meat. See each piece separately.

Lamb neck★★/*Collet d'agneau*: piece of lamb meat to boil or to simmer. Red meat.

Lamb rib★★/*Côte d'agneau*: anterior part of the lamb. Red meat.

Lamb shoulder★★/*Palette d'agneau*: lamb shoulder blade and the flesh around it. Red meat.

Lamb's lettuce★★★/*Mâche*: vegetable plant from which we eat the leaves in salad. Green vegetable.

Lamb stew with beans★/*Haricot de mouton*: lamb stew with dried beans or java beans.
Note: many commercially prepared foods are high in salt: prepare it yourself without salt and with authorized foods.

Lamb sweetbread★★★/*Ris d'agneau*: lamb thymus. Offal.

Lamprey★★★/*Lamproie*: fish with white flesh found in rivers.

Lanark blue: raw or pasteurised sheep's milk cheese. Dairy product.

Lancashire cheese: pasteurised cow's milk cheese. Dairy product.

Langres cheese/*Langres*: soft and fermented cow's milk cheese.

Langue de chat biscuit/*Langue-de-chat*: small plain cookie in the shape of a rounded tongue.

Lapsang souchong★★★/*Souchong*: Chinese black tea. *Note: do not drink it sweetened.*

Lard(1)/*Larder*: prick a meat with small pieces of bacon.

Lard(2)★★★/*Saindoux*: pork fat.

Larded (meat)★★★/*Entrelardée (viande)*: slice of meat relatively fat.

Largemouth bass★★★/*Black-Bass*: fatty freshwater fish.

Lasagna★★/*Lasagne(1)*: dish made of pasta, tomato sauce, ground beef meat and bechamel sauce baked in the oven. Carbohydrate.
Note: many commercially prepared foods are high in salt: prepare it yourself without salt and with authorized foods.

Lasagna sheet★★★/*Lasagne(2)*: pasta in the shape of large flat patches. Carbohydrate.

Lathyrus sativus★★★/*Gesse commune*: vegetable plant from which we eat the cooked seeds. Green vegetable.

Leaf cabbage/*Chou kale*: cf. "Kale".

Lean fish★★★/*Poisson maigre*: fish with white flesh, moderately rich in polyunsaturated fats and in omega 3: sole, cod, pollock, gurnard, carp, roach, pike, zander, etc.
Note: do not consume salted and/or smoked fish. A few lean fish are ★★. Cook it without fat and salt: en papillote, in water, grill, roast...

Lean fish fillet★★★/*Filet de poisson maigre*: slice of fish with white flesh in general without fishbone.
Note: do not consume salted and/or smoked fish. A few lean fish fillet are ★★. Cook it without fat and salt: en papillote, in water, grill, roast...

Lean (meat or fish)★★★/*Maigre (viande ou poisson)*: meat or fish containing very low quantities of fat.

Leaven★★★/*Levain*: piece of batter being fermented mixed to bread batter to make it rise and ferment it.

Leek★★★/*Poireau*: vegetable plant entirely edible. Green vegetable.

Leek seed★★★/*Graine de poireau*: leek seed eaten crushed or germinated.

Leg of deer★★/Gigue: deer leg. Game. Red meat.

Lemon balm★★★/*Mélisse*: aromatic plant used as a condiment.

Lemon curd/*Crème de citron*: spread made of butter, sugar and lemon.

Lemon in light syrup★/*Citron au sirop léger*: poached lemon preserved in more or less sugary water.

Lemon in syrup/*Citron au sirop*: poached lemon preserved in sugary water.

Lemon juice★★★/*Jus de citron*: juice made of the pressing of lemons.

Lemonade/*Citronnade*: beverage made of lemon juice and sugary water.

Lemongrass★★★/*Citronnelle*: grass used as an aromatic plant.

Lemon soda/*Limonade*: fizzy beverage made of sugar, lemon essence and carbon dioxide.

Lentil★★★/*Lentille*: annual plant grown for its seeds which are dried legumes. Carbohydrate.

Lentil flake★★★/*Flocon de lentille*: small portion of dehydrated lentil. Carbohydrate. Gluten-free.

Lentil flour★★★/*Farine de lentille*: powder made of lentil milling. Gluten-free.

Lentil pasta★★★/*Pâte alimentaire de lentille*: mix to be cooked made of lentil flour. Carbohydrate. Gluten-free.

Lesser sand eel★★★/*Equille*: small and elongated saltwater fish with white flesh.

Lettuce★★★/*Laitue*: annual vegetable plant eaten in salad. Green vegetable.

Licorice/*Réglisse*: small confection aniseed-flavored.

Liederkranz cheese: cow's milk cheese with pasteurized milk. Dairy product.

Light fruit compote★/*Compote de fruit allégée*: mix of fresh or dried fruits cooked with a little bit of water and added sugar.
Note: consume it immediately after the meal.

Light iced tea★★★/*Thé glacé light*: infusion of sweetened tea in bottle drunk fresh, sugar-free.

Light industrial ready-cooked dishes/*Plat cuisiné industriel light*: various low-fat dishes sold vacuum packed, frozen or fresh, industrially made and ready to be eaten.

Light industrial vinaigrette sauce/*Sauce vinaigrette industrielle allégée*: sauce industrially made of vegetable oil and vinegar and containing low quantities of fats.

Lightly salted butter/*Beurre demi-sel allégé*: salted dietary fats made from the cream of cow's milk.

Lightly salted margarine/*Margarine demi-sel allégée*: salted plant-based dietary fats.

Light mayonnaise/*Mayonnaise allégée*: cold sauce made of an emulsion of egg yolks, mustard and oil reduced in fats.

Light sirup★★★/sirop 0% de sucre: solution made of water and Sweetener (no sugar).

Light soda★★★/*Soda light*: fizzy beverage made of water, gas and one or several sweetener(s).

Lima bean/*Haricot de lima*: cf. "Fava bean".

Lincolnshire poacher: cow's milk cheese with raw milk. Dairy product.

Ling★★★/*Lingue*: saltwater fish with white flesh.

Linseed oil★★★/*Huile de lin*: fatty substance made of linseeds.

Liqueur★/*Liqueur*: strong alcoholic beverage.
Note: do not drink alcoholic beverage, however no problem if it's cooked.

Liquid sterilized UHT cream (from 3,2% to 5% fats)★★★/*Crème stérilisée liquide UHT (de 3,2% à 5% de matières grasses)*: fats from the milk (3,2% to 5%) sterilized with which the butter is made. Made of sterilized UHT milk. Dairy product.

Liquid sterilized UHT cream (from 12% to 15% fats)★★★/*Crème stérilisée liquide UHT (de 12% à 15% de matières grasses)*: fats from the milk (12% to 15%) sterilized with which the butter is made. Made of sterilized UHT milk. Dairy product.

Little tunny★★★/*Thonine*: fatty saltwater fish.

Livarot cheese/*Livarot*: soft cow's milk cheese with washed rind. Dairy product.

Liver mousse/*Mousse de foie*: cooked meat made of emulsified liver.

Lobster/*Homard*: sea crustacean appreciated for its delicate flesh.

Loin of veal★★★/*Rouelle de veau*: thick slice of veal leg.

Lollipop/*Sucette*: candy made of sugar fixed on a stick. Fast-acting sugar.

Longan in light syrup★/*Longane au sirop léger*: poached longan preserved in more or less sugary water. Exotic fruit.

Longan in syrup/*Longane au sirop*: poached longan preserved in very sugary water. Exotic fruit.

Lovage★★★/*Livèche*: plant from which we eat the seeds and the fresh leaves. Green vegetable.

Low-fat cow's milk cheese★/*Fromage de vache allégé en matières grasses*: cheese made of partly skimmed cow's milk. Dairy product.
Note: almost all cheeses are too salty.

Low-fat fromage blanc★★★/*Fromage blanc allégé en matières grasses*: fresh cheese a bit drained and not aged which contains less fat than usual. Dairy product.

Low-fat goat milk cheese★/*Fromage de chèvre allégé en matières grasses*: cheese made of partly skimmed goat milk. Dairy product.
Note: almost all cheeses are too salty.

Low-fat industrial ready-cooked dishes/*Plat cuisiné industriel allégé en matières grasses*: cf. "Light industrial ready-cooked dishes".

Low-fat margarine★★/*Margarine allégée en matières grasses*: low-fat plant-based dietary fats.
Note: only if it's unsalted.

Low-fat petit suisse★★★/*Petit-suisse allégé en matières grasses*: fromage frais in cylindrical shape made of skimmed milk. Dairy product.

Low-fat pie crust★★/*Pâte brisée allégée en matières grasses*: crust made of flour, low-fat butter and eggs. Carbohydrate.
Note: many commercially prepared foods are high in salt: prepare it yourself without salt and with authorized foods.

Low-fat puff pastry★★/*Pâte feuilletée allégée en matières grasses*: pastry made of flour, low-fat butter and eggs. Carbohydrate.
Note: many commercially prepared foods are high in salt: prepare it yourself without salt and with authorized foods.

Low-fat sheep cheese★/*Fromage de brebis allégé en matières grasses*: cheese made of partly skimmed sheep cheese. Dairy product.
Note: almost all cheeses are too salty.

Low-fat sweet shortcrust pastry★★/*Pâte sablée allégée en matières grasses*: pastry made of flour, low-fat butter, sugar and eggs. Carbohydrate.
Note: many commercially prepared foods are high in salt and/or in sugar so prepare it yourself without salt and sugar and with authorized foods.

Low-salt food/*Allégé en sel*: a food containing a lower quantity of salt than the original food.

Low-sodium★★★/*Hyposodé*: is said about foods containing low quantities of sodium, so low in salt.

Low-sodium ham/*Jambon blanc à teneur réduite en sel*: boneless pork ham cooked in a low-sodium stock. Cooked meat.

Low-sugar breakfast cookie/*Biscuit pour petit-déjeuner allégé en sucre*: cookie adapted to breakfast, rich in cereals and low in sugar. Carbohydrate.

Low-sugar food★★★/*Allégé en sucre*: a food containing a lower quantity of sugar than the original food.

Low-sugar jam/*Confiture allégée en sucre*: jam which sugar quantity is reduced compared to original jam.

Lucerne seed★★★/*Graine de luzerne*: alfalfa seed eaten crushed or germinated.

Lumpfish roe/*Œuf de lumps*: red or black fish eggs.

Lupin flour★★★/*Farine de lupin*: powder made of lupin seeds milling. Gluten-free.

Lupin milk★★/*Lait de lupin*: plant milk from lupin seeds. Lactose-free.
Note: do not consume it sweetened.

Lupin milk cream dessert/*Crème dessert au lait de lupin*: vegetable dessert made of lupin milk, sugar and eggs. Dairy product.

Lychee in light syrup★/*Litchi au sirop léger*: poached lychee preserved in more or less sugary water. Exotic fruit.

Lychee in syrup/*Litchi au sirop*: poached lychee preserved in very sugary water. Exotic fruit.

Lychee juice/*Jus de litchi*: juice made of the pressing of lychees. Exotic fruit.

M

Maasdam cheese★★/*Maasdam*: hard cow's milk cheese.
Note: consume it in moderation, no more than 1 oz per day of autorized cheese.

Macadamia nut/*Noix de macadamia*: cf. "Nut".

Macadamia nut spread/*Pâte à tartiner de noix de macadamia*: very sugary and fat mix of crushed macadamia nuts.

Macaroni★★★/*Macaroni*: hard wheat semolina pasta in the shape of a tube. Carbohydrate.

Macaroon/*Macaron*: small soft round cake made of almonds, white eggs and sugar.

Macchiato★★/*Café noisette*: coffee with a drop of milk.
Note: do not drink it sweetened.

Mace★★★/*Macis*: capsule and peel of the nutmeg used as a condiment.

Macédoine★★★/*Macédoine*: mix of green vegetables or fruits cut in pieces.
Note: do not eat canned vegetables (unless low in salt).

Mackerel in muscadet wine/*Maquereau au muscadet*: preserved mackerel fillets marinated in muscadet wine.

Mackerel in white wine/*Maquereau au vin blanc*: preserved mackerel fillets marinated in dry white wine.

Mackerel rillettes/*Rillettes de maquereau*: cooked meat made of mackerel cooked in vegetable oil.

Mackerel with escabeche sauce/*Maquereau à la sauce escabèche*: mackerel fillets preserved in escabeche sauce.

Mackerel with lemon/*Maquereau au citron*: mackerel fillets preserved in lemon.

Mackerel with mustard sauce/*Maquereau à la moutarde*: mackerel fillets preserved in mustard sauce.

Mackerel with tomato sauce/*Maquereau à la sauce tomate*: mackerel fillets preserved in tomato sauce.

Madeira wine★/*Madère*: fortified wine.
Note: do not drink alcoholic beverage, however no problem if it's cooked.

Madeira wine sauce★★/*Sauce madère*: sauce made of flour, butter, lardons, stock and Madeira wine.
Note: many commercially prepared foods are high in salt: prepare it yourself without salt and with authorized foods.

Madeleine/*Madeleine*: small cake in the shape of a bulging shell.

Malted yeast/Levure maltée: yeast made of barley malt.

Mandarin in light syrup★/*Mandarine au sirop léger*: poached mandarin preserved in more or less sugary water.

Mandarin in syrup/*Mandarine au sirop*: poached mandarin preserved in very sugary water.

Mandarin juice/*Jus de mandarine*: juice made of the pressing of mandarins.

Mango in light syrup★/*Mangue au sirop léger*: poached mango preserved in more or less sugary water. Exotic fruit.

Mango in syrup/*Mangue au sirop*: poached mango preserved in very sugary water. Exotic fruit.

Mango juice/*Jus de mangue*: juice made of the pressing of mangoes. Exotic fruit.

Maple syrup/*Sirop d'érable*: sweetened solution made from the evaporation of the sugar maple sap.

Maranta arundinacea★★★/*Arrow-root*: starch of Maranta root. Gluten-free.

Mare's milk★★★/*Lait de jument*: whole milk produced by mares.

Margarine★★/*Margarine*: plant-based dietary fats.
Note: only if it's unsalted.

Marinade★★/*Marinade*: liquid aromatic mix made of vinegar, spices, etc. in which meat or fish macerates.
Note: many commercially prepared foods are high in salt: prepare it yourself without salt and with authorized foods.

116

Mariniere (mussels)/*Marinière (moules à la)*: mussels cooked in dry white wine with onions and herbs.

Marinière sauce★★/*Sauce marinière*: white sauce made of fish stock and white wine.
Note: many commercially prepared foods are high in salt: prepare it yourself without salt and with authorized foods.

Marmalade/*Marmelade*: mashed fruits previously cut in pieces and cooked with sugar until they become a purée.

Maroilles cheese/*Maroilles*: soft raw cow's milk cheese with washed rind. Dairy product.

Marshmallow(1)/*Guimauve*: candy with a squishy consistency made of mallow root.

Marshmallow(2)/*Marshmallow*: soft marshmallow coated with powdered sugar and starch.

Mascarpone/*Mascarpone*: very creamy and fresh Italian cheese made of cow's milk. Dairy product.

Maté★★★/*Maté*: herbal tea made of roasted American holly leaves.
Note: do not drink it sweetened.

Mayonnaise★★/*Mayonnaise*: cold sauce made of an emulsion of egg yolks, mustard and oil.
Note: many commercially prepared foods are high in salt: prepare it yourself without salt and with authorized foods.

Mead/*Hydromel*: alcoholic beverage made of honey fermented in water.

Meagre★★★/*Maigre*: saltwater fish with white flesh.

Meat extracts/*Extraits de viande*: beef or poultry meat concentrate in small packet or in cube (like KUB OR).

Meat jelly/*Gelée de viande*: cleared and hardened meat juice.

Meat juice★★★/*Jus de viande*: juice made thanks to the cooking of a meat or of a poultry.

Meatloaf★★/*Pain de viande*: dish made of potatoes, meat, butter and eggs served cold with a mayonnaise.
Note: many commercially prepared foods are high in salt: prepare it yourself without salt and with authorized foods.

Meatloaf pâté en croûte★★/*Pâté de viande en croûte*: dish made of ground meat wrapped in puff pastry. Cooked meat.
Note: many commercially prepared foods are high in salt: prepare it yourself without salt and with authorized foods.

Medlar in light syrup★/*Nèfle au sirop léger*: poached medlar preserved in more or less sugary water.

Medlar in syrup/*Nèfle au sirop*: poached medlar preserved in very sugary water.

Melon in light syrup★/*Melon au sirop léger*: poached melon preserved in more or less sugary water.

Melon in syrup/*Melon au sirop*: poached melon preserved in very sugary water.

Melted cheese/*Fromage fondu*: cheese made of one or two cheese which have been melted. Dairy product. American cheese, cup cheese, Philadelphia ...

Merguez/*Merguez*: fresh spicy sausage made of beef or beef and mutton. Cooked meat.

Meringue/*Meringue*: light pastry made of whipped egg whites and sugar baked in the oven.

Mesclun★★★/*Mesclun*: mix of various young salads and aromatic plants. Green vegetable.

Mesembryanthemum crystallinum★★★**/Ficoïde glaciale**: vegetable plant from which we eat the leaves. Green vegetable.

Mexican sauce★★**/Sauce mexicaine**: sauce made of tomatoes, bell peppers, onions and spices.
Note: many commercially prepared foods are high in salt: prepare it yourself without salt and with authorized foods.

Milanese (fish)★★**/Milanaise (poisson à la)**: fish which has been breaded with an egg before being fried.
Note: many commercially prepared foods are high in salt: prepare it yourself without salt and with authorized foods.

Milanese (meat)★★**/Milanaise (viande à la)**: meat which has been breaded with an egg before being fried.
Note: many commercially prepared foods are high in salt: prepare it yourself without salt and with authorized foods.

Milk chocolate/Chocolat au lait: cocoa powder mixed with sugar and butter or other things (or not)...

Milk in tube/Lait en tube: cf. "Sweetened concentrated milk".

Milk roll/Pain au lait: viennoiserie.

Mille-feuille/Mille-feuille: puff pastry cake stuffed with pastry cream.

Millet flake★★★**/Flocon de millet**: small portion of dehydrated millet. Carbohydrate. Gluten-free.

Millet milk★★**/Lait de millet**: plant milk from millets. Lactose-free.
Note: do not consume it sweetened.

Millet milk cream dessert/Crème dessert au lait de millet: vegetable dessert made of millet milk, sugar and eggs. Dairy product.

Millet pasta★★★/*Pâte alimentaire de millet*: mix to be cooked made of refined millet flour. Carbohydrate. Gluten-free.

Milliasse★★/*Milliasse*: mash made of sieved corn flour before being cooled and grilled. Carbohydrate. Gluten-free.
Note: many commercially prepared foods are high in salt: prepare it yourself without salt and with authorized foods.

Mimolette cheese/*Mimolette*: hard cow's milk cheese. Dairy product.

Miner's lettuce: cf. "Claytonia perfoliata".

Minestrone★★/*Minestrone*: soup made of vegetables and lard with pasta or rice.
Note: many commercially prepared foods are high in salt: prepare it yourself without salt and with authorized foods.

Mint★★★/*Menthe*: aromatic plant used as a condiment.

Mirabelle plum in light syrup★/*Mirabelle au sirop léger*: poached mirabelle plum preserved in more or less sugary water.

Mirabelle plum in syrup/*Mirabelle au sirop*: poached mirabelle plum preserved in very sugary water.

Miso/*Miso*: traditional Japanese dish made of fermented soybean paste.

Mixed vegetables★★★/*Jardinière de légumes*: mix of various green vegetables and carbohydrates cut in small pieces.
Note: do not eat canned vegetables (unless low in salt).

Mocha cake/*Moka*: cake made of a genoise stuffed with a butter cream flavored with coffee.

Mombins in light syrup★/*Mombin au sirop léger*: poached mombins preserved in more or less sugary water. Exotic fruit.

Mombins in syrup/*Mombin au sirop*: poached mombins preserved in very sugary water. Exotic fruit.

Monkey bread★★/*Pain de singe*: fruit from the baobab tree. Exotic fruit.
Note: consume it immediately after the meal.

Monosodium glutamate / *Glutamate monosodique*: glutamate sodium used as a flavor enhancer.

Monterey Jack cheese: pasteurised cow's milk cheese. Dairy product.

Morbier cheese/*Morbier*: pressed raw cow's milk cheese. Dairy product.

Mornay sauce★/*Sauce Mornay*: white sauce to which grated gruyère is added.
Note: many commercially prepared foods are high in salt: prepare it yourself without salt and with authorized foods.

Morsel★/*Bouchée*: puff pastry stuffed with various food compositions, example: bouchée à la reine.
Note: many commercially prepared foods are high in salt: prepare it yourself without salt and with authorized foods.

Moussaka★★/*Moussaka*: dish made of alternating layers of eggplant, ground mutton and thick béchamel baked in the oven.
Note: many commercially prepared foods are high in salt: prepare it yourself without salt and with authorized foods.

Mousseline★★/*Mousseline*: very light mashed potatoes. Carbohydrate.
Note: many commercially prepared foods are high in salt: prepare it yourself without salt.

Mozzarella/*Mozzarella*: soft cow's milk cheese, sometimes made with buffalo's milk. Dairy product.

Muenster cheese: pasteurised cow's milk cheese. Dairy product.

Muesli with dark chocolate/*Muesli au chocolat noir*: mix of cereal flakes and dark chocolate curls. Carbohydrate.

Muesli with dried fruits/*Muesli aux fruits secs*: mix of cereal flakes and dried fruits. Carbohydrate.

Muesli with milk chocolate/*Muesli au chocolat au lait*: mix of cereal flakes and milk chocolate curls. Carbohydrate.

Muesli with nuts/*Muesli aux noix*: mix of cereal flakes and various nuts. Carbohydrate.

Muffin(1)/*Muffin(1)*: small plain white bread with leaven. Carbohydrate.

Muffin(2)/*Muffin(2)*: small round cake often containing fruits, sometimes with chocolate.

Mulberries in light syrup★/*Mulberries au sirop léger*: poached mulberries preserved in more or less sugary water.

Mulberries in syrup/*Mulberries au sirop*: poached mulberries preserved in very sugary water.

Mullet★★★/*Mulet*: saltwater and freshwater fish with white flesh.

Multi-grain bread/*Pain multicéréale*: cf. "Wholewheat bread". Carbohydrate.

Multivitamin juice/*Jus multivitaminé*: mix of fruit juices, mainly apple and orange juices.

Mung bean/*Haricot mungo*: cf. "Soy bean".

Mung bean sprout★★★/*Pousse de haricot mungo*: young mung bean sprouts. Green vegetable.

Munster cheese/*Munster*: soft cow's milk cheese with washed rind. Dairy product.

Mushroom in brine/*Champignon en saumure*: sterilized mushroom in its salty cooking water. Green vegetable.

Mushroom sauce★★/*Sauce champignon*: sauce made of tomatoes, onions, mushrooms and herbs.
Note: many commercially prepared foods are high in salt: prepare it yourself without salt and with authorized foods.

Mushroom stock★★/*Fumet de champignon*: very reduced stock made of mushrooms.
Note: many commercially prepared foods are high in salt: prepare it yourself without salt and with authorized foods.

Mussel/*Moule*: edible mollusk.

Mustard/*Moutarde*: condiment made of mustard seeds and vinegar.

Mustard seed★★★/*Graine de moutarde*: mustard seed eaten crushed or germinated.

Myrciaria in light syrup★/*Camu-camu au sirop léger*: poached myrciaria preserved in more or less sugary water. Exotic fruit.

Myrciaria in syrup/*Camu-camu au sirop*: poached myrciaria preserved in very sugary water. Exotic fruit.

$\mathcal{N}$

Nattō/*Nattō*: fermented soy bean sprouts.

Natural apple/*Pomme au naturel*: cf. "Fresh apple".

Natural apricot/*Abricot au naturel*: cf. "Fresh apricot".

Natural aronia/*Aronia au naturel* : cf. "Fresh aronia".

Natural azerole/*Azerole au naturel*: cf. "Fresh azerole".

Natural blackberry/*Mûre au naturel*: cf. "Fresh blackberry".

Natural blackcurrant/*Cassis au naturel*: cf. "Fresh blackcurrant".

Natural button mangosteen/*Mangoustan au naturel*: cf. "Fresh button mangosteen".

Natural carambola/*Carambole au naturel*: cf. "Fresh carambola".

Natural cherimoya/*Anone au naturel*: cf. "Fresh cherimoya".

Natural cherry/*Cerise au naturel*: cf. "Fresh cherry".

Natural clementine/*Clémentine au naturel*: cf. "Fresh clementine".

Natural cranberry/*Canneberge au naturel*: cf. "Fresh cranberry".

Natural fruit cocktail★★/*Cocktail de fruit au naturel*: mix of various fruits cut in dices and preserved in their juice without anything else added.
Note: consume it immediately after the meal.

Natural grapefruit/*Pamplemousse au naturel*: cf. "Fresh grapefruit".

Natural guava/*Goyave au naturel*: cf. "Fresh guava".

Natural jujube/*Jujube au naturel*: cf. "Fresh jujube". Exotic fruit.

Natural kaki/*Kaki au naturel*: cf. "Fresh kaki".

Natural kiwi/*Kiwi au naturel*: cf. "Fresh kiwi".

Natural kumquat/*Kumquat au naturel*: cf. "Fresh kumquat".

Natural lemon/*Citron au naturel*: cf. "Fresh lemon".

Natural longan/*Longane au naturel*: cf. "Fresh longan".

Natural lychee/*Litchi au naturel*: cf. "Fresh lychee".

Natural mandarin/*Mandarine au naturel*: cf. "Fresh mandarin".

Natural mango/*Mangue au naturel*: cf. "Fresh mango".

Natural medlar/*Nèfle au naturel*: cf. "Fresh medlar".

Natural melon/*Melon au naturel*: cf. "Fresh melon".

Natural mirabelle plum/*Mirabelle au naturel*: cf. "Fresh mirabelle plum".

125

Natural mombins/*Mombin au naturel*: cf. "Fresh mombins".

Natural mulberries/*Mulberries au naturel*: cf. "Fresh mulberries".

Natural mushroom★★★/*Champignon au naturel*: sterilized mushroom in its unsalted cooking water. Green vegetable.

Natural myrciaria dubia/*Camu-camu au naturel*: cf. "Fresh myrciaria dubia".

Natural nectarine/*Brugnon au naturel*: cf. "Fresh nectarine".

Natural olive★★★/*Olive au naturel*: fresh olive sterilized in unsalted water.

Natural orange/*Orange au naturel*: cf. "Fresh orange".

Natural papaya/*Papaye au naturel*: cf. "Fresh papaya".

Natural passion fruit/*Grenadille au naturel*: cf. "Fresh passion fruit".

Natural peach/*Pêche au naturel*: cf. "Fresh peach".

Natural pear/*Poire au naturel*: cf. "Fresh pear".

Natural pineapple/*Ananas au naturel*: cf. "Fresh pineapple".

Natural plum/*Prune au naturel*: cf. "Fresh plum".

Natural quince/*Coing au naturel*: cf. "Fresh quince".

Natural rambutan/*Ramboutan au naturel*: cf. "Fresh rambutan".

Natural redcurrant/*Groseille au naturel*: cf. "Fresh redcurrant".

Natural salak/*Salacca au naturel*: cf. "Fresh salak".

Natural salmon/*Saumon au naturel*: salmon preserved without being transformed, except for sterilization, nor without adding anything.

Natural sapodilla fruit/*Sapotille au naturel*: cf. "Fresh sapodilla fruit".

Natural sardine/*Sardine au naturel*: sardine preserved without adding anything nor transforming it, expect for sterilization.

Natural sloe/*Prunelle au naturel*: cf. "Fresh sloe".

Natural sorb/*Sorbe au naturel*: cf. "Fresh sorb".

Natural sweet wine/*Vin doux naturel*: wine fortified thanks to the adding of alcohol during its alcoholic fermentation.

Natural tamarind fruit/*Tamarin au naturel*: cf. "Fresh tamarind".

Natural tuna/*Thon au naturel*: tuna in a can without anything else except for salt.

Natural watermelon/*Pastèque au naturel*: cf. "Fresh watermelon".

Nature knuckle of ham/*Jambonneau nature*: part of the leg above the knee.

Nature shoyu/*Shoyu nature*: fermented soy bean sauce.

Navy bean★★/*Haricot blanc*: white or white and black bean seed eaten fully ripe. Carbohydrate.
Note: do not eat canned navy bean (unless low in salt).

Navy beans with tomato sauce★★/*Haricots blancs sauce tomate*: navy beans cooked in tomato sauce.
Note: many commercially prepared foods are high in salt: prepare it yourself without salt and with authorized foods.

Neapolitan sauce★★/*Sauce napolitaine*: sauce made of tomatoes, olives and various aromatic herbs.
Note: many commercially prepared foods are high in salt: prepare it yourself without salt and with authorized foods.

Nectarine/*Nectarine*: cf. "Peach".

Nectarine in light syrup★/*Brugnon au sirop léger*: poached nectarine preserved in more or less sugary water.

Nectarine in syrup/*Brugnon au sirop*: poached nectarine preserved in very sugary water.

Nettle★★★/*Ortie*: herbaceous plant from which we eat the leaves. Green vegetable.

Neufchâtel cheese★★/*Neufchâtel*: soft cow's milk cheese with bloomy rind. Dairy product.
Note: consume it in moderation, no more than 1 oz per day of autorized cheese.

New Zealand spinach★★★/*Tétragone*: vegetable plant from which we eat the leaves. Green vegetable.

Ninespine stickleback★★★/*Epinochette*: small freshwater fish with white flesh.

Niolo/*Niolo*: goat or sheep milk cheese. Dairy product.

Noisette potato/*Pomme noisette*: dish in the shape of a small ball made of mashed potatoes and flour before being fried and baked in the oven. Carbohydrate.

Nori★★★/*Nori*: edible seaweed.

Nougat/*Nougat*: confection made of a mix of sugar, honey, egg whites, almonds, hazelnuts and pistachios.

Nuoc-mâm sauce/*Sauce nuoc-mâm*: putrefied anchovy extract.

Nutmeg★★★/*Noix de muscade*: fruit from the myristica fragrans which grated seed is used as a condiment.

Nutsedge flake★★★/*Flocon de souchet*: small portion of dehydrated nutsedge. Carbohydrate.

Nutsedge flour★★★/*Farine de souchet*: powder made of nutsedge milling. Gluten-free.

O

Oat bran★★★/*Son d'avoine*: residue of oat milling.

Oat cream★★★/*Crème d'avoine*: more or less liquid cream made of oat milk, substitute to crème fraîche.

Oat flake★★★/*Flocon d'avoine*: small portion of dehydrated oats. Carbohydrate.

Oatmeal★★/*Porridge*: oats mush. Carbohydrate.
Note: many commercially prepared foods are high in salt and/or in sugar so prepare it yourself without salt and sugar and with authorized foods.

Oat milk★★/*Lait d'avoine*: plant milk from oats. Lactose-free.
Note: do not consume it sweetened.

Oat milk cream dessert/*Crème dessert au lait d'avoine*: vegetable dessert made of oat milk, sugar and eggs. Dairy product.

Oat pasta★★★/*Pâte alimentaire à base d'avoine*: mix to be cooked made of refined oat flour. Carbohydrate.

Oats★★★/*Avoine*: cereal which seeds are edible. Carbohydrate.

Octopus/*Poulpe*: octopus from which we eat the tentacles.

Œuf au lait★★/*Œuf au lait*: dessert made of eggs, milk and sugar.
Note: many commercially prepared foods are high in sugar, so prepare it yourself without sugar and with authorized foods.

Offals/*Abats*: edible part of meat animals that is not flesh nor muscles: kidney, liver, tongue, trotter, lungs, blood and black sausage... (See each offal separately in this book).

Okra★★★/*Gombo*: tropical green vegetable.
Note: do not eat canned vegetables (unless low in salt).

Oleaginous fruit★★★/*Fruit oléagineux*: fruit rich in fats, most of the time, it consists in seeds: almonds, nuts, avocados, etc.
Note: only if it's unsalted.

Olive à la grecque/*Olive à la grecque*: olive preserved in a mixture rich in salt and in various spices.

Olive in brine/*Olive en saumure*: fresh olive sterilized in salted water.

Olivet cheese/*Olivet*: soft cow's milk cheese with washed rind. Dairy product.

100% pure juice freshly pressed fruit juice (any fruit)/*Jus de fruit 100% pur jus fraîchement pressé (tous fruits confondus)*: juice made of the pressing of fruits, without adding any sugar or additive (colorant, flavor, preserver...) and drunk immediately.

100% pure juice freshly pressed vegetable juice (any green vegetable)/*Jus de légume 100% pur jus fraîchement pressé (tous légumes verts confondus)*: juice of green vegetables made of the pressing of vegetables, without adding anything and drunk immediately.

100% pure juice industrial fruit juice (any fruit)★★★/*Jus de fruit 100% pur jus industriel (tous fruits confondus)*: fruit juice industrially made of the pressing of fruits, without adding any sugar or additive (colorant, flavor, preserver...).
Note: do not drink tomato juice.

100% pure juice industrial vegetable juice (any green vegetable)/*Jus de légume 100% pur jus industriel (tous légumes verts confondus)*: juice of green vegetables industrially made of the pressing of vegetables without adding anything.

100% whole-grain almond pasta★★★/*Pâte alimentaire à base d'amande complet*: mix to be cooked made of whole-grain almond flour. Gluten-free.

100% whole-grain amaranth pasta★★★/*Pâte alimentaire à base d'amarante complet*: mix to be cooked made of whole-grain amaranth flour. Gluten-free.

100% whole-grain barley pasta★★★/*Pâte alimentaire d'orge complet*: mix to be cooked made of whole-grain barley flour. Carbohydrate.

100% whole-grain buckwheat pasta★★★/*Pâte alimentaire de sarrasin complet*: mix to be cooked made of whole-grain buckwheat flour. Carbohydrate.

100% whole-grain corn pasta
- 100% whole-grain soybean pasta

100% whole-grain corn pasta★★★/*Pâte alimentaire de maïs complet*: mix to be cooked made of whole-grain corn flour. Carbohydrate. Gluten-free.

100% whole-grain einkorn wheat pasta★★★/*Pâte alimentaire de petit épeautre complet*: mix to be cooked made of whole-grain einkorn wheat flour. Carbohydrate.

100% whole-grain findi pasta★★★/*Pâte alimentaire de fonio complet* : mix to be cooked made of whole-grain findi flour. Carbohydrate. Gluten-free.

100% whole-grain khorasan wheat pasta★★★/*Pâte alimentaire de kamut complet*: mix to be cooked made of whole-grain khorasan wheat. Carbohydrate.

100% whole-grain millet pasta★★★/*Pâte alimentaire de millet compet*: mix to be cooked made of whole-grain millet flour. Carbohydrate. Gluten-free.

100% whole-grain oat pasta★★★/*Pâte alimentaire à base d'avoine compet*: mix to be cooked made of whole-grain oat flour. Carbohydrate.

100% whole-grain quinoa pasta★★★/*Pâte alimentaire de quinoa complet*: mix to be cooked made of whole-grain quinoa flour. Carbohydrate. Gluten-free.

100% whole-grain rice pasta★★★/*Pâte alimentaire de riz complet*: mix to be cooked made of whole-grain rice flour. Carbohydrate. Gluten-free.

100% whole-grain rye pasta★★★/*Pâte alimentaire de seigle complet*: mix to be cooked made of whole-grain rye flour. Carbohydrate.

100% whole-grain soybean pasta★★★/*Pâte alimentaire de soja complet*: mix to be cooked made of whole-grain soybean flour. Carbohydrate. Gluten-free.

100% whole-grain spelt pasta★★★/*Pâte alimentaire d'épeautre complet*: mix to be cooked made of whole-grain spelt flour. Carbohydrate.

100% wholewheat pasta★★★/*Pâte alimentaire de blé complet*: mix to be cooked made of wholewheat semolina. Carbohydrate.

Omelet★★★/*Omelette*: dish made of beaten eggs cooked in a frying pan.

Onion★★★/*Oignon*: vegetable plant from which we eat the bulb. Green vegetable.

Onion salt/*Sel d'oignon*: mix of table salt and dehydrated onion in powder.

Onion sausage/*Saucisse à l'oignon*: ground pork flesh seasoned with onions, etc. before being put in a casing made of intestines. Cooked meat.

Onion seed★★★/*Graine d'oignon*: onion seed eaten crushed or germinated.

Oolong tea★★★/*Thé oolong*: tea between green tea and black tea.
Note: do not drink it sweetened.

Orangeade/*Orangeade*: beverage made of orange juice, sugar and water.

Orange in light syrup★/*Orange au sirop léger*: poached orange preserved in more or less sugary water.

Orange in syrup/*Orange au sirop*: poached orange preserved in very sugary water.

Orange juice/*Jus d'orange*: juice made of the pressing of oranges.

Orange roughy★★★/*Empereur*: saltwater fish with white flesh.

Oregano★★★/*Origan*: aromatic plant used as a condiment.

Oriental borage★★★/*Bourrache orientale*: plant used as a condiment and from which we eat the young leaves.

Orzo★★★/*Café d'orge*: drink made of roasted barley malt.
Note: do not drink it sweetened.

Ossau-Iraty/*Ossau-Iraty*: pressed sheep milk cheese.

Osso buco★★/*Osso-buco*: knuckle of veal cut in slices, stir-fried and cooked in a mixture made of dry white wine, onions and tomatoes.
Note: many commercially prepared foods are high in salt: prepare it yourself without salt and with authorized foods.

Ostrich★★★/*Autruche*: big bird living in Africa and in the Middle-East.

Outside flat cut★★/*Gîte à la noix*: posterior part of the leg of beef. Red meat.

Oven fries★★★/*Frites au four*: pre-cooked potatoes not spiced baked in the oven. Carbohydrate. Gluten-free.
Note: only if it's unsalted.

Oxalis tuberosa★★★/*Oca du Pérou*: vegetable plant from which we eat the tubers. Green vegetable.

Ox tripe/*Gras-double*: tripe shop product made of beef rumen. Offal.

Oyster/*Huître*: edible mollusk.

Oyster sauce/*Sauce d'huître*: sauce made of oyster stock reduction with corn starch.

$\mathcal{P}$

Paddy rice/*Riz paddy*: cf. "Whole-grain rice".

Paella/*Paella*: Spanish dish made of rice flavored with saffron, browned in oil and cooked in stock, with meat, fish, crustacea, etc.

Pain au chocolat/*Pain au chocolat*: pastry stuffed with a chocolate bar.

Pain aux raisins/*Pain aux raisins*: viennoiserie made of raisins and custard.

Pain de Gênes/*Pain de Gênes*: viennoiserie made of cookie dough in which crushed almonds are put.

Paleleaved: cf. "Helianthus strumosus".

Palm heart★★/*Cœur de palmier*: edible heart of palm in light brine.
Note: do not eat canned vegetables (unless low in salt).

Palm kernel oil★★★/*Huile de palmiste*: cf. "Palm oil".

Palm oil★★★/*Huile de palme*: fatty substance made of palm kernel.

Palm oil-free margarine★★/*Margarine sans huile de palme*: palm oil-free plant-based dietary fats.
Note: only if it's unsalted.

Pancakes★★/*Pancakes*: small thick crepes made of sieved flour. Carbohydrate.
Note: many commercially prepared foods are high in salt and/or in sugar so prepare it yourself without salt and sugar and with authorized foods.

Pancetta/*Pancetta*: Italian cooked meat made of salted pork breast which has been rolled and dried.

Panettone/*Panettone*: brioche stuffed with dried and candied fruits. Carbohydrate.

Panna cotta/*Panna cotta*: dessert made of milk, sugar, crème fraîche and gelatin.

Papaya in light syrup★/*Papaye au sirop léger*: poached papaya preserved in more or less sugary water. Exotic fruit.

Papaya in syrup/*Papaye au sirop*: poached papaya preserved in very sugary water. Exotic fruit.

Papaya juice/*Jus de papaye*: juice made of the pressing of papayas. Exotic fruit.

Paprika★★★/*Paprika*: sweet chili pepper in powder.

Paraffin oil★★★/*Huile de paraffine*: vegetable oil that is not assimilated by your metabolism.

Parmesan cheese/*Parmesan*: hard Italian cheese made of cow's milk. Dairy product.

Parsley★★★/Persil: vegetable plant used as a condiment. Green vegetable.

Parsley juice★★/*Jus de persil*: juice made of the pressing of parsley.
Note: many commercially prepared foods are high in salt: prepare it yourself without salt.

Parsley seed★★★/***Graine de persil***: parsley seed eaten crushed or germinated.

Parsnip★★★/***Panais***: vegetable plant grown for its edible root. Green vegetable.

Parsnip chips/*Chips de panais*: very thinly cut parsnip, fried and salted.

Partridge★★★/***Perdrix***: edible and very appreciated bird. Game.

Passion fruit in light syrup★/***Grenadille au sirop léger***: poached passion fruit preserved in more or less sugary water. Exotic fruit.

Passion fruit in syrup/*Grenadille au sirop*: poached passion fruit preserved in very sugary water. Exotic fruit.

Passion fruit juice/Jus de fruit de la passion: juice made of the pressing of passion fruits. Exotic fruit.

Pasteurized milk★★★/***Lait pasteurisé***: milk which has been thermally treated between 160°F and 185°F during 15 seconds before being rapidly cooled.

Paupiette/*Paupiette*: slice of meat stuffed with stuffing wrapped around itself. Made of pork, turkey or veal.

Pea milk★★/***Lait de pois***: plant milk from peas. Lactose-free.
Note: do not consume it sweetened.

Pea milk cream dessert/*Crème dessert au lait de pois*: vegetable dessert made of pea milk, sugar and eggs. Dairy product.

Peach in light syrup★/***Pêche au sirop léger***: poached peach preserved in more or less sugary water.

Peach in syrup/*Pêche au sirop*: poached peach preserved in very sugary water.

Peach juice/*Jus de pêche*: juice made of the pressing of peaches.

Peanut★★/*Cacahuète*: roasted seed of the peanut plant. *Note: only if it's unsalted.*

Peanut butter/*Beurre de cacahuète*: peanut mixed with sugar.

Peanut flour★★★/*Farine d'arachide*: powder made of not wholewheat peanut milling. Gluten-free.

Peanut milk★★/*Lait d'arachide*: plant milk from peanuts. Lactose-free.
Note: do not consume it sweetened.

Peanut oil★★★/*Huile d'arachide*: fatty substance made of peanut.

Peanut purée★★★/*Purée d'arachide*: mashed peanut seeds to spread.

Pear in light syrup★/*Poire au sirop léger*: poached pear preserved in more or less sugary water.

Pear in syrup/*Poire au sirop*: poached pear preserved in very sugary water.

Pear juice/*Jus de poire*: juice made of the pressing of pears.

Pecan nut/*Noix de pécan*: cf. "Nut".

Peking duck/*Laqué (canard)*: duck which has been coated with sweet and sour sauce between two cookings.

Pecking pork/*Laqué (porc)*: pork which has been coated with sweet and sour sauce between two cookings.

Pepino dulce★★★/*Poire-melon*: annual vegetable plant producing this fruit.

Pepper★★★/*Poivre*: greatly savory and spicy spice.

Pepper sauce★★/*Sauce au poivre*: sauce made with flour and butter with milled pepper.
Note: many commercially prepared foods are high in salt: prepare it yourself without salt and with authorized foods.

Perch★★★/*Perche*: freshwater fish with white flesh.

Pesto/*Pesto*: mix of ground basil, garlic, grated parmesan cheese and olive oil.

Pesto sauce/*Sauce pesto*: sauce made of tomatoes, basils and parmesan cheese.

Petit four/*Petit-four*: small pastry the size of a morsel, made of a dry pastry or stuffed with cream.

Petit suisse★★★/*Petit-suisse*: fromage frais in cylindrical shape. Dairy product.

Petit suisse flavored with fruits/*Petit-suisse aromatisé aux fruits*: sweetened fromage frais in cylindrical shape with fruits. Dairy product.

Pheasant★★★/*Faisan*: gallinaceous bird valued for its flesh. Game.

Philadelphia cheese: pasteurised cow's milk cheese. Dairy product.

Physalis peruviana★★★/*Coqueret du Pérou*: vegetable plant from which we eat the berries.

Pickle/*Cornichon*: kind of cucumber harvested young or very young and preserved in vinegar or brine. Green vegetable.

Pickles★★★/*Pickles*: small vegetables or fruits preserved in vinegar.
Note: many commercially prepared foods are high in salt: prepare it yourself without salt and with authorized foods.

Pickleweed/*Salicorne*: plant found on sea shores and from which we eat the stems as a condiment. Green vegetable.

Picodon/*Picodon*: soft raw goat milk cheese.

Pie★★/*Tarte*: dish made of a thick pie garnished with cream, fish, meat, etc. before being baked in the oven.
Note: many commercially prepared foods are high in salt: prepare it yourself without salt and with authorized foods.

Pie crust★★/*Pâte brisée*: crust made of flour, butter and eggs. Carbohydrate.
Note: many commercially prepared foods are high in salt: prepare it yourself without salt and with authorized foods.

Pig's ear★★★/*Oreille de cochon*: pork's ear. Offal.

Pigeon★★★/*Pigeon*: small edible bird. Game.

Pike★★★/*Brochet*: freshwater fish with white flesh.

Pineapple in light syrup★/*Ananas au sirop léger*: poached pineapple preserved in more or less sugary water. Exotic fruit.

Pineapple in syrup/*Ananas au sirop*: poached pineapple preserved in very sugary water. Exotic fruit.

Pineapple juice/*Jus d'ananas*: juice made of the pressing of pineapples. Exotic fruit.

Pine kernel★★★/*Pignon de pin*: crushed pine kernel.

Pink grapefruit juice/*Jus de pamplemousse rose*: juice made of the pressing of pink grapefruits.

Pinto bean★★★/*Haricot rosé*: cooked pinky seed eaten fully ripe. Carbohydrate.

Piperade★/*Piperade*: dish made of bell pepper, tomatoes and eggs.
Note: many commercially prepared foods are high in salt: prepare it yourself without salt and with authorized foods.

Pistachio★★★/*Pistache*: seed from the pistachio tree.
Note: only if it's unsalted.

Pistachio cream★★★/*Crème de pistache*: pistachio spread.

Pistachio milk★★/Lait de pistache: plant milk from pistachios. Lactose-free.
Note: do not consume it sweetened.

Pistachio milk cream dessert/*Crème dessert au lait de pistache*: vegetable dessert made of pistachio milk, sugar and eggs. Dairy product.

Pistachio purée★★★/*Purée de pistache*: mashed pistachios to spread.

Pitta/Pita: small unleavened white bread. Carbohydrate.

Pizza★/*Pizza*: bread dough galette covered with tomato sauce and various garnishes before being baked in the pizza oven. Carbohydrate.
Note: many commercially prepared foods are high in salt: prepare it yourself without salt and with authorized foods.

Pizza base★★/*Pâte à pizza*: base made of flour, water and yeast.
Note: many commercially prepared foods are high in salt: prepare it yourself without salt.

Plaice★★★/*Carrelet*: flat saltwater fish with white flesh.

141

Plain breast bacon
- Plain whole goat milk yogurt

Plain breast bacon★★★/*Lard de poitrine nature*:
plain piece of pork breast.

Plain cookie/*Biscuit sec*: cookie made of flour, sugar,
eggs and fats.

Plain lardon★★★/*Lardon nature*: small piece of plain
bacon used to prepare a dish.

Plain skimmed cow's milk yogurt★★★/*Yaourt au
lait de vache maigre nature*: cow's milk which has
been partially or completely skimmed before being
fermented thanks to lactic acid bacteria, unsweetened.
Dairy product.

Plain skimmed goat milk yogurt★★★/*Yaourt au
lait de chèvre maigre nature*: goat milk which has been
partially or completely skimmed before being fermented
thanks to lactic acid bacteria, unsweetened. Dairy product.

Plain skimmed sheep milk yogurt★★★/*Yaourt au
lait de brebis maigre nature*: sheep milk which has
been partially or completely skimmed before being
fermented thanks to lactic acid bacteria, unsweetened.
Dairy product.

**Plain sweetened whole cow's milk
yogurt**★★★/*Yaourt au lait de vache entier nature
sucré*: whole cow's milk fermented thanks to lactic acid
bacteria before being sweetened. Dairy product.

Plain whole cow's milk yogurt★★★/*Yaourt au lait
de vache entier nature*: whole cow's milk fermented
thanks to lactic acid bacteria, unsweetened. Dairy product.

Plain whole goat milk yogurt★★★/*Yaourt au lait
de chèvre entier nature*: whole goat milk fermented
thanks to lactic acid bacteria, unsweetened. Dairy product.

Plain whole sheep milk yogurt★★★/*Yaourt au lait de brebis entier nature*: whole sheep milk fermented thanks to lactic acid bacteria, unsweetened. Dairy product.

Plantain★★★/*Banane plantain*: tropical fruit of the banana tree, rich in starch and eaten cooked. Exotic fruit.

Planter's punch/Planteur: punch made of rum, cane sugar and fruit juice.

Plant milk/*Lait végétal*: milk from various vegetables. All are lactose-free. See each plant milk separately.

Plum in light syrup★/*Prune au sirop léger*: poached plum preserved in more or less sugary water.

Plum in syrup/*Prune au sirop*: poached plum preserved in very sugary water.

Polenta(1)★★/*Polenta(1)*: chestnut mush. Gluten-free. *Note: many commercially prepared foods are high in salt: prepare it yourself without salt and with authorized foods.*

Polenta(2)★★★/*Polenta(2)*: corn mush. Gluten-free.

Pont-L'évêque cheese/*Pont-L'évêque*: soft cow's milk with washed rind. Dairy product.

Popcorn/*Maïs pop corn*: puffed up corn kernel more or less sweetened. Gluten-free.

Poppy seed★★★/*Graine de pavot*: poppy seed eaten crushed.

Poppyseed oil★★★/*Huile d'œillette*: fatty substance made of poppy seeds.

Porgy★★★/*Sar*: saltwater fish with white flesh.

Pork (meat...)/*Porc (viande de...)*: all unprepared nor transformed meats, plain, ready to be cooked and cut from pork. See each piece separately.

Pork breast★★★/*Poitrine de porc*: inferior part of the pork's rib cage to boil.

Pork chop★★★/*Côte de porc*: anterior part of the pork.

Pork confit★★/*Confit de porc*: pork cooked and preserved in its cooking fat.
Note: many commercially prepared foods are high in salt: prepare it yourself without salt and with authorized foods.

Pork hotpot★★/*Potée*: dish made of pork meat and boiled cabbage.
Note: many commercially prepared foods are high in salt: prepare it yourself without salt and with authorized foods.

Pork kidney★★/*Rognon de porc*: kidney of the pork. Offal.

Pork liver★★★/*Foie de porc*: offal.

Pork liver pâté/*Pâté de foie de porc*: minced pork liver cooked before being put in a baking pan. Cooked meat.

Pork loin(1)★★★/*Echine de porc*: anterior part of the pork.

Pork loin(2)★★★/*Longe de porc*: pork meat corresponding to the upper part of the cervical and lumbar areas.

Pork loin(3)★★★/*Rouelle de porc*: thick slice of pork leg.

Pork rillettes/*Rillettes de porc*: cooked meat made of pork meat cooked in its fat.

Pork shoulder★★★/*Palette de porc*: pork shoulder blade and the flesh around it.

Pork spare ribs★★★/*Carré de porc*: piece of pork meat to roast or to grill.

Pork tongue★★★/*Langue de porc*: pork tongue eaten boiled. Offal.

Porridge★★★/*Bouillie*: doughy dish made of boiled flour and milk, or water. Carbohydrate.
Note: do not consume it sweetened.

Port salut/*Port-salut*: pressed cow's milk cheese with washed rind. Dairy product.

Port wine/*Porto*: liqueur wine.

Potato★★★/*Pomme de terre*: vegetable plant from which we eat the tubers. Carbohydrate. Gluten-free.

Potatoes chips/*Chips de pomme de terre*: very thinly cut potatoes, fried and salted.

Potato flake/*Flocon de pommes de terre*: small portion of dehydrated potato, to make purée. Carbohydrate. Gluten-free.

Potato flakes purée/*Purée de pomme de terre en flocon*: dehydrated industrial mashed potatoes.

Potato starch★★★/*Fécule de pomme de terre*: starch from potatoes transformed into flour. Carbohydrate. Gluten-free.

Pot-au-feu★★/*Pot-au-feu*: dish made of boiled beef meat, carrots, leeks, cabbage... Red meat.
Note: many commercially prepared foods are high in salt: prepare it yourself without salt and with authorized foods.

Poulette sauce★★/*Sauce poulette*: white sauce with egg yolks and lemon juice.
Note: many commercially prepared foods are high in salt: prepare it yourself without salt and with authorized foods.

Pouligny Saint-Pierre cheese★★/*Pouligny Saint-Pierre*: raw goat milk cheese in the shape of a pyramid.
Note: consume it in moderation, no more than 1 oz per day of autorized cheese.

Poultry★★★/*Volaille*: bird raised in barnyard such as hens, chickens, ducks, guinea fowls, gooses etc.

Poultry liver/*Foie de volaille*: chicken, hen, duck, goose, etc. offal.

Poultry liver pâté/*Pâté de foie de volaille*: minced poultry liver cooked before being put in a baking pan. Cooked meat.

Poultry quenelle/*Quenelle de volaille*: poultry stuffing thickened with eggs and bread crumb before being shaped in the form of a sausage.

Poultry sausage/*Saucisse de volaille*: sausage made of poultry meat. Cooked meat.

Poultry stock★★/*Fond de volaille*: brown stock made of poultry stock.
Note: many commercially prepared foods are high in salt: prepare it yourself without salt and with authorized foods.

Pout★★★/*Tacaud*: saltwater fish with white flesh.

Powder of dehydrated broth/*Bouillon déshydraté en poudre*: cf. "Cube of... broth".

Powder of myrciaria★★★/*Camu-camu en poudre*: extracts of myrciaria sold in capsules or in powder. Exotic fruit.

Powdered sugar/*Sucre glace*: white sugar in extremely thin powder. Fast-acting sugar.

Praline(1)/*Pralin*: mix of roasted and crushed hazelnuts and almonds with sugar.

Praline(2)/*Praliné*: mix of chocolate and crushed sugared almonds.

Preserve★/*Conserve*: sterilized food preserved in an airtight can.
Note: do not consume unless it's unsalted or/and no sweetened.

Preserved plain grilled mackerel/*Maquereau grillé nature en conserve*: preserved plain grilled mackerel fillets.

Pressed cooked cheese★/*Fromage à pâte pressée cuite*: beaufort cheese, comté cheese, emmental cheese, gruyère, parmesan cheese, capricious, Colby, Swiss cheese, Dry Jack... Dairy product.
Note: almost all cheeses are too salty.

Pressed uncooked cheese★/*Fromage à pâte pressée non cuite*: appenzeller cheese, cantal cheese, cheddar, édam cheese, Humboldt fog...
Note: almost all cheeses are too salty.

Pretzel/*Bretzel*: cookie into an 8-shape, sprinkled with salt and cumin.

Prickly pear★★/*Figue de Barbarie*: plump fruit from the opuntia (cactus).
Note: consume it immediately after the meal.

Prickly pear juice/*Jus de figue de Barbarie*: juice made of the pressing of prickly pears.

Prime rib of beef★★★/*Côte de bœuf*: piece of beef meat to grill.

Provel cheese
- Puffed einkorn wheat pancake

Provel cheese: pasteurised cow's milk cheese. Dairy product.

Provençale sauce★★/*Sauce provençale*: sauce made of tomatoes, onions, bell peppers, olives, olive oil and thyme.
Note: many commercially prepared foods are high in salt: prepare it yourself without salt and with authorized foods.

Provolone/*Provolone*: cow's milk cheese which has been salted, dried and smoked. Dairy product.

Prune/*Pruneau*: plum which has been dried in the oven or to the sun.

Prune juice/*Jus de pruneau*: juice made of the pressing of prunes.

Pudding/*Pudding*: sugary dessert made of bread crumb, semolina or rice, plain cookie, eggs, crème fraîche and dried fruits.

Puffed barley pancake/*Galette d'orge soufflée*: extruded barley pancake. Carbohydrate. Gluten-free.

Puffed buckwheat pancake/*Galette de sarrasin soufflé*: extruded buckwheat pancake. Carbohydrate.

Puffed chocolate rice pancake/*Galette de riz soufflé au chocolat*: extruded white rice pancake coated with chocolate. Gluten-free.

Puffed corn pancake/*Galette de maïs soufflé*: extruded corn pancake. Carbohydrate. Gluten-free.

Puffed einkorn wheat pancake/*Galette de petit épeautre soufflé*: extruded einkorn wheat pancake. Carbohydrate.

Puffed einkorn whole-grain pancake/*Galette de petit épeautre complet soufflé*: extruded whole-grain einkorn wheat pancake. Carbohydrate.

Puffed khorasan wheat pancake/Galette de kamut soufflé: extruded khorasan wheat pancake. Carbohydrate. Gluten-free.

Puffed millet pancake/*Galette de millet soufflé*: extruded millet pancake. Carbohydrate. Gluten-free.

Puffed oats pancake/*Galette d'avoine soufflée*: extruded oats pancake. Carbohydrate. Gluten-free.

Puffed quinoa pancake/*Galette de quinoa soufflé*: extruded quinoa pancake. Carbohydrate.

Puffed rice pancake/*Galette de riz soufflé*: extruded rice pancake. Carbohydrate. Gluten-free.

Puffed rye pancake/*Galette de seigle soufflé*: extruded rye pancake. Carbohydrate. Gluten-free.

Puffed soybean pancake/*Galette de soja soufflé*: extruded soybean pancake. Carbohydrate. Gluten-free.

Puffed spelt pancake/*Galette d'épeautre soufflé*: extruded spelt pancake. Carbohydrate.

Puffed whole-grain barley pancake/*Galette d'orge complète soufflée*: extruded whole-grain barley pancake. Carbohydrate. Gluten-free.

Puffed whole-grain buckwheat pancake/*Galette de sarrasin complet soufflé*: extruded whole-grain buckwheat pancake. Carbohydrate.

Puffed whole-grain corn pancake/*Galette de maïs complet soufflé*: extruded whole-grain corn pancake. Carbohydrate. Gluten-free.

Puffed whole-grain khorasan wheat pancake - Pumpkin

Puffed whole-grain khorasan wheat pancake/*Galette de kamut complet soufflé*: extruded whole-grain khorasan wheat pancake. Carbohydrate. Gluten-free.

Puffed whole-grain millet pancake/*Galette de millet complet soufflé*: extruded whole-grain millet pancake. Carbohydrate. Gluten-free.

Puffed whole-grain oats pancake/*Galette d'avoine complète soufflée*: extruded whole-grain oat pancake. Carbohydrate. Gluten-free.

Puffed whole-grain rice pancake/*Galette de riz complet soufflé*: extruded whole-grain rice pancake. Carbohydrate. Gluten-free.

Puffed whole-grain rye pancake/*Galette de seigle complet soufflé*: extruded whole-grain rye pancake. Carbohydrate. Gluten-free.

Puffed whole-grain soybean pancake/*Galette de soja complet soufflé*: extruded whole-grain soybean pancake. Carbohydrate. Gluten-free.

Puffed whole-grain spelt pancake/*Galette d'épeautre complet soufflé*: extruded whole-grain spelt pancake. Carbohydrate.

Puff pastry★★/*Pâte feuilletée*: pastry made of flour, butter and eggs. Carbohydrate.
Note: many commercially prepared foods are high in salt: prepare it yourself without salt and with authorized foods.

Pulp-free fruit juice/*Jus de fruit sans pulpe*: 100% pure juice fruit juice without the pulp.

Pumpkin(1)★★★/*Citrouille*: kind of squash, very big autumn fruit. Green vegetable.

Pumpkin(2)★★★/*Potiron*: vegetable plant from which we eat the fruit. Green vegetable.

Pumpkin seed flour★★★/*Farine de pépin de courge*: powder from pumpkin seed milling. Gluten-free.

Punch/*Punch*: alcoholic beverage made of rum and fruit juice.

Purée★★/*Purée*: dish made of mashed green vegetables or some mashed carbohydrates.
Note: many commercially prepared foods are high in salt: prepare it yourself without salt and with authorized foods.

Purslane★★★/*Pourpier*: plant from which we eat the leaves in salad. Green vegetable.

Purslane seed★★★/*Graine de pourpier*: purslane seed eaten crushed or germinated.

Q

Quail★★★/*Caille*: small migratory bird close to the partridge. Game.

Queen coris pâté/*Pâte de tamarin*: pressed and concentrated queen coris.

Quiche★★/*Quiche*: salted pie made of pie crust and garnished with lardons covered with flan mixture: eggs and crème fraîche.
Note: many commercially prepared foods are high in salt: prepare it yourself without salt and with authorized foods.

Quince in light syrup★/*Coing au sirop léger*: poached quince preserved in more or less sugary water.

Quince in syrup/*Coing au sirop*: poached quince preserved in very sugary water.

Quince jelly/*Pâte de coing*: confection made of quinces cooked in sugar.

Quinoa★★★/*Quinoa*: plant from which we eat the seeds. Carbohydrate. Gluten-free.

Quinoa cornflakes/*Corn flakes de quinoa*: grilled flakes made of quinoa flour. Carbohydrate. Gluten-free.

Quinoa cream★★★/*Crème de quinoa*: more or less liquid cream made of quinoa milk, substitute to crème fraîche.

Quinoa flake★★★/*Flocon de quinoa*: small portion of dehydrated quinoa. Carbohydrate. Gluten-free.

Quinoa flour★★★/*Farine de quinoa*: powder made of not whole-grain quinoa seed milling. Carbohydrate. Gluten-free.

Quinoa milk★★/*Lait de quinoa*: plant milk from quinoa. Lactose-free.
Note: do not consume it sweetened.

Quinoa milk cream dessert/*Crème dessert au lait de quinoa*: vegetable dessert made of quinoa milk, sugar and eggs. Dairy product.

Quinoa pasta★★★/*Pâte alimentaire de quinoa*: mix to be cooked made of refined quinoa flour. Carbohydrate. Gluten-free.

Quinoa seed★★★/*Graine de quinoa*: quinoa seed eaten crushed or germinated.

Quinoa tabbouleh★★/*Taboulé de quinoa*: mix of quinoa, tomatoes, onions, bell peppers, raisins and mint leaves with olive oil. Carbohydrate. Gluten-free.
Note: many commercially prepared foods are high in salt: prepare it yourself without salt and with authorized foods.

ℛ

Rabbit terrine/Pâté de lapin: minced rabbit meat cooked before being put in a baking pan. Cooked meat.

Rabbit★★/*Lapin*: herbivore mammal.

Raclette(1)/*Raclette(1)*: cow's milk cheese eaten melted. Dairy product.

Raclette(2)/*Raclette(2)*: dish made of raclette cheese, potatoes and various cooked meats.

Radish★★★/*Radis*: vegetable plant from which we eat the plump root. Green vegetable.

Raisin/*Raisin sec*: fruit from the vine which has been greatly dried.

Ramaria aurea★★★/*Clavaire doré*: mushroom you can find in the woods. Green vegetable.

Rambutan in light syrup★/*Ramboutan au sirop léger*: poached rambutan preserved in more or less sugary water. Exotic fruit.

Rambutan in syrup/*Ramboutan au sirop*: poached rambutan preserved in very sugary water. Exotic fruit.

Rampion bellflower★★★/*Raiponce cultivée*: vegetable plant grown for its leaves and its roots eaten in salad. Green vegetable.

Rare (cooking)
- Ready-to-use flour for white bread

Rare (cooking)★★/*Saignante (cuisson)*: to not completely cook beef, duck or lamb. Red meat.

Raspberry juice/*Jus de framboise*: juice made of the pressing of raspberries.

Ratatouille★★/*Ratatouille*: dish made of eggplants, bell peppers, tomatoes and zucchinis.
Note: many commercially prepared foods are high in salt: prepare it yourself without salt and with authorized foods.

Raviole/*Raviole*: small square of pasta stuffed with cheese. Carbohydrate.

Raw (raw milk, raw meat, raw fish...)★★★/*Cru (lait cru, viande crue, poisson cru...)*: food eaten without being previously cooked.

Raw milk★★★/*Lait cru*: milk from animals not thermally treated nor filtered.

Raw milk cheese★/*Fromage au lait cru*: cheese made of milk that did not go under any heat treatment. Dairy product.
Note: almost all cheeses are too salty.

Razor clam/*Couteau*: sea mollusk with a long shell.

Ready-cooked dishes from the caterer/*Plat cuisiné du traiteur*: various dishes sold vacuum packed, frozen or fresh, made by an artisan from catering profession and ready to be eaten.

Ready-to-use flour for cereal bread/*Farine pour pain aux céréales prête à l'emploi*: whole-grain cereal flour with seeds and salt.

Ready-to-use flour for white bread/*Farine pour pain blanc prête à l'emploi*: salted sieved cereal flour.

Ready-to-use flour for wholewheat bread/Farine pour pain complet prête à l'emploi: salted whole-grain cereal flour.

Reblochon/*Reblochon*: pressed raw cow's milk cheese with a washed rind. Dairy product.

Red ascophyllum/*Goémon rouge*: edible seaweed.

Red berries fruit/*Jus de fruits rouges*: juice made of the pressing of red berries.

Redcurrant in light syrup★/*Groseille au sirop léger*: poached redcurrant preserved in more or less sugary water.

Redcurrant in syrup/*Groseille au sirop*: poached redcurrant preserved in very sugary water.

Red hawk cheese: pasteurised cow's milk cheese. Dairy product.

Red kuri squash★★★/*Potimarron*: squash which taste is similar to that of the chestnut. Green vegetable.

Red Leicester cheese: raw or pasteurised cow's milk cheese. Dairy product.

Red meat★★/*Viande rouge*: beef, lamb and horse meat.

Red mullet★★★/*Rouget*: saltwater fish with white flesh.

Red rice★★★/*Riz rouge*: rare red whole-grain rice.

Red sea bream★★★/*Rousseau*: saltwater fish with white flesh.

Red wine★/*Vin rouge*: wine made thanks to the alcoholic fermentation of black grapes under the action of yeasts.
Note: do not drink alcoholic beverage, however no problem if it's cooked.

Red windsor: pasteurised cow's milk cheese. Dairy product.

Red yeast rice★★★/*Levure de riz rouge*: microscopic mushrooms grown on rice.

Reindeer milk★★★/*Lait de renne*: whole milk produced by reindeers.

Remoulade sauce★★/*Sauce rémoulade*: sauce made of vegetable oil, mustard and shallots.
Note: many commercially prepared foods are high in salt: prepare it yourself without salt and with authorized foods.

Rhubarb★★★/*Rhubarbe*: vegetable plant from which we eat the chards after cooking. Green vegetable.
Note: do not eat canned vegetables (unless low in salt).

Rib steak★★/*Entrecôte*: slice of beef cut between the ribs. Red meat.

Rice bran★★★/*Son de riz*: residue of rice milling.

Rice bran oil★★★/*Huile de riz*: fatty substance made of rice.

Rice bulgur★★★/*Boulgour de riz*: crushed white rice steamed or cooked in water. Carbohydrate. Gluten-free.

Rice cornflakes/*Corn flakes de riz*: grilled flakes made of white rice flakes. Carbohydrate. Gluten-free.

Rice cream★★★/*Crème de riz*: more or less liquid cream made of rice milk, substitute to crème fraîche.

Rice flake★★★/*Flocon de riz*: small portion of dehydrated rice. Carbohydrate. Gluten-free.

Rice flour★★★/*Farine de riz*: powder made of white rice milling. Carbohydrate. Gluten-free.

Rice milk★★/*Lait de riz*: plant milk from rice. Lactose-free.
Note: do not consume it sweetened.

Rice milk cream dessert/*Crème dessert au lait de riz*: vegetable dessert made of rice milk, sugar and eggs. Dairy product.

Rice milk yogurt★★/*Yaourt au lait de riz*: rice milk fermented thanks to lactic acid bacteria, sweetened or not. Dairy product. Lactose-free.
Note: do not consume it sweetened.

Rice pasta★★★/*Pâte alimentaire de riz*: mix to be cooked made of refined rice flour. Carbohydrate. Gluten-free.

Rice syrup/*Sirop de riz*: sweetener made from the fermentation of grain of rice and barley.

Ricotta★★/*Ricotta*: Italian cheese made of other cheese serum. Dairy product.

Rigotte/*Rigotte*: raw goat milk cheese and raw cow's milk cheese. Dairy product.

Rind★★★/*Couenne*: pork skin.

Rind (cheese)★/*Croûte (du fromage)*: external part of the cheese.
Note: almost all cheeses are too salty.

Risotto★★/*Risotto*: rice cooked in broth with onions and various other foods.
Note: many commercially prepared foods are high in salt: prepare it yourself without salt and with authorized foods.

Roach★★★/*Gardon*: freshwater fish with white flesh.

Roast★★★/*Rôti*: piece of meat or of poultry baked in the oven.

Roast beef★★/*Rosbif*: piece of roasted beef. Red meat.

Roasted spelt★★★/*Epeautre torréfié*: roasted beverage similar to coffee.
Note: do not drink it sweetened.

Rocamadour cheese★★/*Rocamadour*: round and flat cheese made of raw goat milk. Dairy product.
Note: consume it in moderation, no more than 1 oz per day of authorized cheese.

Rockfish★★★/*Sébaste*: saltwater fish with white flesh.

Rognonnade/*Rognonnade*: veal loin rolled and garnished with kidneys. Offal.

Rollmops/*Rollmops*: raw herring rolled around a pickle marinated in vinegar and spices.

Rollot/*Rollot*: soft cow's milk cheese in the shape of a heart. Dairy product.

Romanesco broccoli★★★/*Chou romanesco*: cabbage from which we eat the central inflorescence.

Rond de tranche★★★/*Rond de tranche*: fat and very tender piece of beef corresponding to quadriceps. Red meat.

Rooster/*Coq*: cf. "Hen". Poultry.

Roquefort/*Roquefort*: raw sheep milk cheese with parsley in it. Dairy product.

Rose hip★★★/*Cynorhodon*: berry from the dog rose eaten as jam.

Rosemary★★★/*Romarin*: aromatic plant.

Rosé wine/*Vin rosé*: pink wine.

Roux★★/Roux: mix of flour and burnt butter used to thicken sauces.
Note: many commercially prepared foods are high in salt: prepare it yourself without salt and with authorized foods.

Royal jelly★★★/*Gelée royale*: liquid secreted by nurse bees.

Ruffe★★★/*Grémille*: small freshwater with white flesh.

Rum★/*Rhum*: eau de vie made from sugar cane juice distillation.
Note: do not drink alcoholic beverage, however no problem if it's cooked.

Rum baba/*Baba*: yeast cake with raisins and soaked with rum or Kirsch after cooking.

Rump steak★★/*Rumsteck*: tender piece of beef to grill or to roast. Red meat.

Rutabaga★★★/*Rutabaga*: vegetable plant from which we eat the swollen root. Green vegetable.
Note: do not eat canned vegetables (unless low in salt).

Rye★★★/*Seigle*: cereal source of gluten from which flour is extracted. Carbohydrate.

Rye bread/*Pain de seigle*: bread made of rye flour. Carbohydrate.

Rye flake★★★/*Flocon de seigle*: small portion of dehydrated rye. Carbohydrate.

Rye milk★★/*Lait de seigle*: plant milk from rye. Lactose-free.
Note: do not consume it sweetened.

Rye milk cream dessert/*Crème dessert au lait de seigle*: vegetable dessert made of rye milk, sugar and eggs. Dairy product.

Rye pasta★★★/*Pâte alimentaire de seigle*: mix to be cooked made of refined rye flour. Carbohydrate.

S

Saccharine★★★/*Saccharine*: synthetic sweetener.

Saccharose/*Saccharose*: cf. "White sugar".

Safflower oil★★★/*Huile de carthame*: fatty substance made of safflower.

Saffron★★★/*Safran*: spice.

Sage★★★/*Sauge*: plant used as a condiment.

Saint-André cheese/*Saint-André*: soft cow's milk cheese with bloomy rind. Triple cream cheese. Dairy product.

Sainte-Maure/*Sainte-Maure*: raw goat milk cheese in the shape of a long cylinder. Dairy product.

Saint-Félicien cheese/*Saint-Félicien*: cf. "Saint-Marcellin".

Saint-Florentin/*Saint-Florentin*: soft raw or pasteurized cow's milk cheese with washed rind. Dairy product.

Saint Honoré cream/*Crème saint honoré*: cf. "Custard". Dairy product.

Saint-Marcellin/*Saint-Marcellin*: soft cow's milk cheese with bloomy rind. Dairy product.

Saint-Nectaire★★/*Saint-Nectaire*: pressed raw cow's milk cheese with bloomy rind. Dairy product.
Note: consume it in moderation, no more than 1 oz per day of authorized cheese.

Saint-Paulin cheese/*Saint-Paulin*: pressed raw cow's milk cheese with washed rind. Dairy product.

Salad★★★/*Salade*: leafy vegetable plant such as watercress, curly endive, lettuce, lamb's lettuce, etc. Green vegetable.

Salad burnet★★★/*Pimprenelle*: aromatic plant used as a condiment.

Salak in light syrup★/*Salacca au sirop léger*: poached salak preserved in more or less sugary water. Exotic fruit.

Salak in syrup/*Salacca au sirop*: poached salak preserved in very sugary water. Exotic fruit.

Salami/*Salami*: Italian saucisson sec. Cooked meat.

Salers cheese/*Salers*: pressed raw cow's milk cheese.

Salmis★★/*Salmis*: stew made of game or poultry pieces cooked in a sauce made of red wine.
Note: many commercially prepared foods are high in salt: prepare it yourself without salt and with authorized foods.

161

Salmon carpaccio★★/*Carpaccio de saumon*: salmon flesh cut in very thin slices eaten raw, with a drop of olive oil and lemon juice.
Note: many commercially prepared foods are high in salt: prepare it yourself without salt and with authorized foods.

Salmon quenelle/*Quenelle de saumon*: salmon stuffing thickened with eggs and bread crumb before being shaped in the form of a sausage.

Salmon rillettes/*Rillettes de saumon*: cooked meat made of salmon cooked in vegetable oil.

Salsify★★/*Salsifis*: vegetable plant from which we eat the root. Green vegetable.
Note: do not eat canned vegetables (unless low in salt).

Salt pork/*Petit salé*: pork breast cooked in a flavored stock.

Salt pork with lentils/*Petit salé aux lentilles*: dish cooked in sauce and made of pork breast and lentils.

Salt-free & gluten-free crispbread★★★/*Biscotte sans sel & sans gluten*: slice of salt-free and gluten-free sandwich bread industrially toasted in the oven. Carbohydrate.

Salt-free cookie/*Biscuit sans sel*: cookie that does not contain salt. Carbohydrate.

Salt-free crispbread★★★/*Biscotte sans sel*: slice of salt-free sandwich bread industrially toasted in the oven. Carbohydrate.

Salt-free grain bread★★★/*Pain aux céréales sans sel*: bread made of wholewheat flour with cereal grains with not salt in the batter during the kneading. Carbohydrate.

Salt-free margarine★★★/*Margarine sans sel*: salt-free plant-based dietary fats.

Salt-free white bread★★★/***Pain blanc sans sel***: bread made of sieved cereal flour with no salt in the batter during the kneading. Carbohydrate.

Salt-free wholewheat bread★★★/***Pain complet sans sel***: bread made of wholewheat flour with no salt in the batter during the kneading. Carbohydrate.

Salt substitute★★★/***Substitut de sel***: preparation without sodium chloride used as a substitute to salt.
Note: ask your doctor if you can consume it!

Saltwater fish★★★/***Poisson marin***: every fatty and lean fish found in salted waters.
Note: do not consume salted and/or smoked fish. A few fish are ★★. Cook it without fat and salt: en papillote, in water, grill, roast...

Samosa/*Samoussa*: triangular fritter made of a thin flour dough wrapping a stuffing made of meat, fish, rice vermicelli, green vegetables, etc.

Sandwich★/***Sandwich***: bread cut in slices between which you put a slice of meat, fish, cheese, etc.
Note: many commercially prepared foods are high in salt: prepare it yourself without salt and with authorized foods.

Sandwich bread/*Pain de mie*: white bread without crust. Carbohydrate.

Sapodilla fruit in light syrup★/***Sapotille au sirop léger***: poached sapodilla fruit preserved in more or less sugary water. Exotic fruit.

Sapodilla fruit in syrup/*Sapotille au sirop*: poached sapodilla fruit preserved in very sugary water. Exotic fruit.

Sardine in chili pepper★★/***Sardine au piment***: sardine preserved in oil and in chili pepper.
Note: only if it's unsalted.

163

Sardine in herbes★★/*Sardine aux herbes*: sardine preserved in oil and aromatic herbes.
Note: only if it's unsalted.

Sardine in lemon★★/*Sardine au citron*: sardine preserved in oil and lemon.
Note: only if it's unsalted.

Sardine in oil★★/*Sardine à l'huile*: sardine preserved in oil.
Note: only if it's unsalted.

Sardine in tomato sauce/*Sardine à la tomate*: sardine preserved in tomato sauce.

Sardinella★★★/*Sardinelle*: fatty saltwater fish.

Sardine rillettes/*Rillettes de sardine*: cooked meat made of sardine cooked in vegetable oil.

Sashimi/*Sashimi*: dish made of raw fish and seafoods with soy sauce.

Sashimi sauce/*Sauce sashimi*: cf. "Sushi sauce".

Sauce gribiche★★/*Sauce gribiche*: sauce made of eggs, vegetable oil, pickles, vinegar and herbs.
Note: many commercially prepared foods are high in salt: prepare it yourself without salt and with authorized foods.

Saucisson sec/*Saucisson sec*: big sausage eaten raw after desiccation. Cooked meat.

Sauerkraut(1)/*Choucroute(1)*: fermented white cabbage.

Sauerkraut(2)/*Choucroute(2)*: fermented white cabbage with cooked meats, pork meat and potatoes.

Sauté (cooking process)★★★/*Sauté (cuisson en)*: to cook food in fat over an open fire.

Savory★★★/*Sarriette*: plant used as a condiment.

Savory cake/*Cake*: cake made of an egg batter with yeast, candied fruits and raisins soaked in rum.

Sbrinz/*Sbrinz*: hard raw cow's milk which has been aged for a long time. Dairy product.

Scabbard fish★★★/*Sabre*: saltwater fish with white flesh.

Scallion★★★/*Ciboule*: plant close to the garlic and from which we eat the bulging leaves.

Scallop★/*Coquille saint Jacques*: edible sea mollusk.

Scolymus★★★/*Scolyme*: vegetable plant from which we eat the roots. Green vegetable.

Scorpion fish★★★/*Rascasse*: saltwater fish with white flesh.

Scorzonera★★/*Scorsonère*: vegetable plant from which we eat the long black roots. Green vegetable.
Note: do not eat canned vegetables (unless low in salt).

Scotch/*Scotch*: Scottish whiskey.

Scrambled egg★★★/*Œuf brouillé*: lightly cooked scrambled egg in an oiled frying pan.

Sculpin★★★/*Chabot*: freshwater fish with white flesh.

Sea bream★★/*Daurade* : saltwater fish with white flesh.

Seafood/*Fruit de mer*: edible crustacea and shellfish. See each of them depending on their own name.

Sea lettuce/*Ulve*: edible seaweed. Green vegetable.

Sea trout★★/*Truite de mer*: fatty saltwater fish.

Sea urchin★/*Oursin*: very thorny saltwater animal.

Seaweed chips/*Chips d'algue*: cooked and compressed seaweeds very thinly cut before being fried and salted.

Seaweed mustard/*Moutarde aux algues*: condiment made of mustard seeds, edible seaweeds and vinegar.

Seaweed tartare/*Tartare d'algue*: dish made of edible seaweeds, vegetable oil and various condiments.

Seeds★★★/*Graines*: mix of sunflower seeds, wheat seeds, barley seeds, sesame seeds, etc.
Note: only if it's unsalted.

Seltz water★★★/*Eau de seltz*: water that is naturally or artificially fizzy.

Semi-skimmed cow's milk★★★/*Lait de vache demi-écrémé*: milk produced by cows and which has been partially skimmed.

Semi-skimmed goat milk★★★/*Lait de chèvre demi-écrémé*: goat milk which has been partially skimmed.

Semi-skimmed sheep milk★★★/*Lait de brebis demi-écrémé*: sheep milk which has been partially skimmed.

Sepiola/*Sépiole*: small edible cuttlefish.

Serviceberry★★/*Alise*: red fruit from the whitebeam.
Note: consume it immediately after the meal.

Sesame cream★★★/*Crème de sésame*: condiment made of crushed sesame seeds.

Sesame flour★★★/*Farine de sésame*: powder made of sesame seeds milling. Gluten-free.

Sesame oil★★★/*Huile de sésame*: fatty substance made of sesame seeds.

Sesame purée★★★/*Purée de sésame*: mashed sesame seeds to spread.

Sesame seed★★★/*Graine de sésame*: sesame seed eaten crushed.

Sesame seed milk★★/*Lait de graines de sésame*: plant milk from sesame seeds. Lactose-free.
Note: do not consume it sweetened.

Sesame seeds milk cream dessert/*Crème dessert au lait de graines de sésame*: vegetable dessert made of sesame seed milk, sugar and eggs. Dairy product.

Shad★★★/*Alose*: fatty freshwater fish.

Shallot★★★/*Echalote*: vegetable plant close to the onion and grown for its bulb. Green vegetable.

Shandy/*Panaché*: beverage made for half of beer and half of lemon soda.

Shashlik★★/*Chachlik*: goat meat skewered and marinated in spicy vinegar. Red meat.
Note: many commercially prepared foods are high in salt: prepare it yourself without salt and with authorized foods.

Sheep milk cheese★/*Fromage de brebis*: cheese made of sheep milk. Dairy product.
Note: almost all cheeses are too salty.

Sheep milk cottage cheese★★★/*Faisselle au lait de brebis*: fresh cheese made of sheep milk. Dairy product.

Sheep milk cream dessert/*Crème dessert au lait de brebis*: dairy specialty or dessert made of sheep milk, sugar and eggs. Dairy product.

Sheep milk fromage blanc
- Shropshire cheese

Sheep milk fromage blanc★★★/*Fromage blanc de brebis*: fresh cheese made of sheep milk, a bit drained and not aged. Dairy product.

Shepherd's pie★★/*Hachis parmentier*: dish made of ground meat and mashed potatoes grilled into the oven.
Note: many commercially prepared foods are high in salt: prepare it yourself without salt and with authorized foods.

Sherry/*Xérès*: cf. "Vinegar".

Shiitake★★★/*Shiitake*:   fresh   or   dried   edible mushroom. Green vegetable.

Shin★★/*Gîte*: beef shank. Red meat.

Shirred egg★★/*Œuf cocotte*: egg with crème fraîche baked in the oven in ramekins.
Note: many commercially prepared foods are high in salt: prepare it yourself without salt and with authorized foods.

Shortbread biscuit/*Sablé*: small round biscuit made of sugar, egg yolks and butter.

Shoulder of beef★★/*Macreuse*: piece of beef made of the shoulder muscles to simmer or to boil. Red meat.

Shoulder of lamb★★/*Epaule d'agneau*: tender and rather fat meat from the lamb. Red meat.

Shoulder of veal★★★/*Epaule de veau*: tender meat to roast coming from the veal.

Shrimp/*Crevette*: small sea crustacean.

Shrimp chips/*Chips de crevette*: swelled chips made of tapioca and shrimp flours.

Shropshire cheese: pasteurised cow's milk cheese. Dairy product.

Sichuan pepper★★★/***Poivre de Sichuan***: spice.

Silurid fish★★★/***Silure***: freshwater fish with white flesh.

Sirloin★★/***Aloyau***: piece of beef meat consisting of the fillet, the sirloin and the rump steak. Red meat.

Sirloin steak★★/***Faux-filet***: tasty but fat beef meat. Red meat.

Sium sisarum★★★/***Chervis***: vegetable plant from which we eat the cooked roots. Green vegetable.

62% fat lightly salted butter/*Beurre demi-sel à 62% de matières grasses*: lightly salted butter which fat quantity has been reduced from one fourth compared to traditional butter.

62% fat lightly unsalted butter★★★/***Beurre doux à 62% de matières grasses***: unsalted butter which fat quantity has been reduced from one fourth compared to traditional butter.

Skate (wing)★/***Raie (aile de)***: gristly saltwater fish. Fish with white flesh.

Skimmed cow's milk★★★/***Lait de vache écrémé***: cow's milk which has been completely skimmed.

Skimmed goat milk★★★/***Lait de chèvre écrémé***: goat milk completely skimmed.

Skipjack tuna★★★/***Bonite***: fatty saltwater fish.

Skirt steak★★/***Hampe de bœuf***: portion of the beef diaphragm. Red meat.

Slice of fillet★★★/***Tranche de filet***: piece of pork meat to grill.

Slippery elm★★★/*Orme rouge*: powder made of slippery elm bark.

Sloe in light syrup★/*Prunelle au sirop léger*: poached sloe preserved in more or less sugary water.

Sloe in syrup/*Prunelle au sirop*: poached sloe preserved in very sugary water.

Small pea★★/*Petit pois*: round and green seed from the pea harvested fresh. Green vegetable.

Smelt★★★/*Eperlan* : saltwater fish with white flesh.

Smoked breast bacon/*Lard de poitrine fumé*: salted and smoked piece of pork breast.

Smoked fatty fish/*Poisson gras fumé*: fatty fish which has been salted (more or less) and smoked.

Smoked haddock/*Haddock*: smoked haddock fish.

Smoked ham/*Jambon fumé*: raw pork ham salted before being smoked. Cooked meat.

Smoked herring/*Hareng fumé*: herring which went under a smoking process.

Smoked lardon/*Lardon fumé*: small piece of salted and smoked bacon used to prepare a dish.

Smoked lean fish/*Poisson maigre fumé*: lean fish which has been salted (more or less) and smoked.

Smoked meat/*Viande fumée*: meat which has been salted before being smoked.

Smoked salmon/*Saumon fumé*: salmon which has been salted before being smoked.

Smoked sausage/*Saucisse fumée*: pork sausage which has been smoked. Cooked meat.

Smoked trout/*Truite fumée*: filet of salted and smoked trout.

Smoked vegetable ham/*Jambon végétal fumé*: vegetarian product made of cereals and vegetable oil.

Snails★★/*Escargot*: small gastropod mollusk.

Snow pea★★★/Pois mange-tout: kind of peas from which we eat the clove and the seeds. Green vegetable.

Soda/*Soda*: fizzy beverage made of water, gas and sugar, or even fruit juice.

Soft-boiled egg★★★/*Œuf à la coque*: egg cooked in a lot of water without the egg yolk being completely cooked.

Soft cheese with bloomy rind★/*Fromage à pâte molle et à croûte fleurie*: brie cheese, camembert, carré de l'Est, chaource cheese, coulommiers cheese, neufchâtel cheese, saint-marcellin, d'Isigny cheese... Dairy product.
Note: almost all cheeses are too salty.

Soft cheese with washed rind★/*Fromage à pâte molle et à croûte lavée*: époisses de Bourgogne, munster cheese, livarot cheese, maroilles cheese, olivet cendré, pont-l'évêque cheese, rollot cheese, saint-florentin cheese, soumaintrain cheese, vacherin cheese, Red hawk, Muenster, Teleme cheese, Brick cheese, lierderkrantz cheese... Dairy product.
Note: almost all cheeses are too salty.

Soft frik★★★/*Frik tendre*: crushed not fully grown hard wheat without its peel. Carbohydrate.

Soft pepper★★★/*Poivre doux*: not very savory and not very spicy spice.

Soft shell clam/*Mye*: shellfish, edible saltwater mollusk.

Sole★/*Sole*: flat saltwater fish with white flesh.

Soluble coffee/*Café soluble*: grains of dehydrated coffee.

Sorbet/*Sorbet*: frozen dessert made of sugar and fruit purée or fruit juice.

Sorbet-filled fruit/*Givré*: fruit which inside part is stuffed with sorbet.

Sorb in syrup/*Sorbe au sirop*: poached sorb preserved in very sugary water.

Sorb preserved in light syrup★/*Sorbe au sirop léger*: poached sorb preserved in more or less sugary water.

Sorghum flake★★★/*Flocon de sorgho*: small portion of dehydrated sorghum. Carbohydrate.

Sorghum flour★★★/*Farine de sorgho*: powder made of sorghum milling. Carbohydrate. Gluten-free.

Sorghum pasta★★★/*Pâte alimentaire de sorgho*: mix to be cooked made of sorghum flour. Carbohydrate. Gluten-free.

Sorrel★★★/*Oseille*: vegetable plant with edible leaves. Green vegetable.

Soufflé★★/*Soufflé*: dish made of whipped egg whites which, during the cooking process, increase the volume of the dish.
Note: many commercially prepared foods are high in salt: prepare it yourself without salt and with authorized foods.

Soumaintrain/*Soumaintrain*: soft cow's milk cheese with a washed rind. Dairy product.

Soursop★★/*Corossol*: fruit from the Annona muricata. Exotic fruit.
Note: consume it immediately after the meal.

Soybean★★★/*Soja*: legume from which we eat the seeds.
Note: do not eat canned vegetables (unless low in salt).

Soy bean★★★/*Haricot de soja*: green soybean seed. Green vegetable.
Note: do not eat canned vegetables (unless low in salt).

Soybean flake★★★/*Flocon de soja*: small portion of dehydrated soybean. Carbohydrate.

Soybean flour★★★/*Farine de soja*: flour made of not whole-grain soybean milling. Gluten-free.

Soybean pasta★★★/*Pâte alimentaire de soja*: mix to be cooked made of refined soybean flour. Carbohydrate. Gluten-free.

Soy bean sprout★★★/*Germe de soja*: young sprout from the mung bean seed. Green vegetable.

Soybean vermicelli★★★/*Vermicelle chinois*: pasta made of soybean flour in the shape of long and thin filaments. Gluten-free.

Soy cream★★★/*Crème de soja*: more or less liquid cream made of soy milk, substitute to crème fraîche.

Soy milk★★/*Lait de soja*: plant milk from soybean. Lactose-free.
Note: do not consume it sweetened.

Soy milk cream dessert/*Crème dessert au lait de soja*: vegetable dessert made of soy milk, sugar and eggs. Dairy product.

Soy milk fromage blanc★★/*Fromage blanc de soja*: fresh cheese made of soy milk. Dairy product. Lactose-free.
Note: do not consume it sweetened.

Soy milk yogurt★★/*Yaourt au lait de soja*: soy milk fermented thanks to lactic acid bacteria, sweetened or not. Dairy product. Lactose-free.
Note: do not consume it sweetened.

Soy oil★★★/*Huile de soja*: fatty substance made of soybean.

Soy sauce/*Sauce soja*: fermented vegetable proteins with meat flavors.

Spare rib★★★/*Travers de porc*: extremity of pork ribs.

Sparkling wine/*Vin mousseux*: wine or cider containing carbon dioxide.

Speculaas/*Spéculoos*: very sugary plain cookie.

Spelt bulgur★★★/*Boulgour d'épeautre*: sieved and crushed spelt steamed or cooked in water. Carbohydrate.

Spelt coffee★★★/*Café d'épeautre*: spelt seeds drunk once roasted.
Note: do not drink it sweetened.

Spelt cornflakes/*Corn flakes d'épeautre*: grilled flakes made of sieved spelt flakes. Carbohydrate.

Spelt flake★★★/*Flocon d'épeautre*: small portion of dehydrated spelt. Carbohydrate.

Spelt milk★★/*Lait d'épeautre*: plant milk from spelts. Lactose-free.
Note: do not consume it sweetened.

Spelt milk cream dessert/*Crème dessert au lait d'épeautre*: vegetable dessert made of spelt milk, sugar and eggs. Dairy product.

Spelt pasta★★★/*Pâte alimentaire d'épeautre*: mix to be cooked made of refined spelt flour. Carbohydrate.

Spices/*Epices*: clove, chili pepper, turmeric, curry, etc. See the different spices separately.

Spider crab/*Araignée*: sea crustacean looking like a crab.

Spiky bitter melon★★★/*Margose à piquant*: vegetable plant from which we eat the green fruits. Green vegetable.

Spinach★★★/*Epinard*: vegetable plant from which we eat the long leaves. Green vegetable.
Note: do not eat canned vegetables (unless low in salt).

Spinach seed★★★/*Graine d'épinard*: spinach seed eaten crushed or germinated.

Spiny dogfish★★★/*Aiguillat*: edible shark.

Spirulina/*Spiruline*: sea cyanobacteria used to make diet foods.

Spirulina pasta/*Pâte alimentaire de spiruline*: mix to be cooked made of spirulina. Green vegetable.

Split pea/*Pois cassé*: dried peas eaten in purée. Carbohydrate. Gluten-free.

Split pea flake/*Flocon de pois cassés*: small portion of dehydrated split pea flakes. Carbohydrate. Gluten-free.

Split pea pasta/*Pâte alimentaire de pois cassés*: mix to be cooked made of split pea flour. Carbohydrate. Gluten-free.

Spring roll/*Nem*: small rice flour crepe stuffed with meat, vegetables and rice vermicelli before being rolled and fried. Gluten-free.

Spring roll sauce/*Sauce pour nem*: cf. "Nuoc-mâm sauce".

Squash seed★★★/*Graine de courge*: grilled squash seed.

Squash seed oil★★★/*Huile de pépin de courge*: fatty substance made of squash seeds.

Squash seed purée★★★/*Purée de graine de courge*: mashed squash seeds to spread.

Squid/*Calamar*: sea mollusk very appreciated for its flesh.

Stachys affinis★★★/*Crosne du Japon*: vegetable plant from which we eat the rhizomes. Green vegetable.

Standard olive oil★★★/*Huile d'olive standard*: fatty substance made of olive.

Star anise/*Anis étoilé*: cf. "Anise".

Steak tartare★★/*Steak tartare*: ground beef steak eaten raw. Red meat.
Note: do not salt.

Steak/*Steak*: cf. "Beefsteak".

Steam★★/*Etouffée (à l')*: cooking method for meats and dried legumes with a very small quantity of liquid or even no liquid at all and a lid on.
Note: many commercially prepared foods are high in salt: prepare it yourself without salt and with authorized foods.

Sterilized UHT heavy cream★★★/*Crème entière stérilisée UHT*: fats from sterilized milk (30%) with which the butter is made. Made of sterilized UHT milk. Dairy product.

Stevia (extracts)★★★/*Stévia (extraits de)*: very sugary extract of a plant called "Stevia", used as a sweetener instead of sugar, very low in calorie.

Stew(1)★★/*Civet*: rabbit or other game stew marinated in red wine and cooked in a sauce thickened with blood. Game.
Note: many commercially prepared foods are high in salt: prepare it yourself without salt and with authorized foods.

Stew(2)★★/*Ragoût*: dish made of meat or fish cut in pieces and cooked in a sauce made of roux.
Note: many commercially prepared foods are high in salt: prepare it yourself without salt and with authorized foods.

Stichelton cheese: raw cow's milk cheese. Dairy product.

Stickleback★★★/*Epinoche*: small freshwater fish with white flesh.

Still water★★★/*Eau plate*: natural water from the faucet or in bottle.

Stilton cheese/*Stilton*: cow's milk cheese with pasteurized milk parsley in it. Dairy product.

Stinking bishop: pasteurised cow's milk cheese. Dairy product.

Stir fry of cooked and frozen green vegetables/*Poêlée de légumes verts cuisinés surgelés*: green vegetables industrially cooked before being frozen and ready to be eaten.

**Stir fry of uncooked frozen green vegetables
-Sugared almond**

Stir fry of uncooked frozen green vegetables★★★**/Poêlée de légumes verts non cuisinés surgelés**: plain green vegetables frozen, sold with their spices packet and ready to be eaten.

Stock★★**/Court bouillon**: flavored liquid in which you cook fish or meat.
Note: many commercially prepared foods are high in salt: prepare it yourself without salt and with authorized foods.

Strawberry juice/Jus de fraise: juice made of the pressing of strawberries.

Strudel/Strudel: pastry made of a rolled pastry stuffed with cinnamon apple and raisin.

Stuffed breakfast cookie/Biscuit pour petit-déjeuner fourré: stuffed cookie adapted to breakfast. Carbohydrate.

Stuffed olive/Olive farcie: olive stuffed with various condiments such as anchovies, bell peppers, etc.

Stuffing★★**/Farce**: mix of mashed herbs, mashed vegetables, ground meat and crushed bread crumb put inside a poultry, a fish or a vegetable.
Note: many commercially prepared foods are high in salt: prepare it yourself without salt and with authorized foods.

Sucralose★★★**/Sucralose**: sweetener used instead of sugar to get a sugary taste, very low in calorie.

Sugar cane/Sucre de canne: sugar only from cane sugar. Fast-acting sugar.

Sugared almond/Dragée: almond, chocolate or nut coated with sugar.

Sugar-free and salt-free cookie★★★/*Gâteau sec sans sucre sans sel*: sugar-free but sweetened (in general with maltitol) cookie which contains a low quantity of salt or even no salt at all.

Sugar-free and semi-skimmed powder cow's milk★★★/*Lait de vache demi-écrémé en poudre sans sucre*: dehydrated semi-skimmed cow's milk without added sugar.

Sugar-free and semi-skimmed powder goat milk★★★/*Lait de chèvre demi-écrémé en poudre sans sucre*: dehydrated semi-skimmed goat milk without added sugar.

Sugar-free and semi-skimmed powder sheep milk★★★/*Lait de brebis demi-écrémé en poudre sans sucre*: dehydrated semi-skimmed sheep milk without added sugar.

Sugar-free cake/*Gâteau sans sucre*: pastry made of a sugar-free but sweetened batter, used alone or with a cream, fruits...

Sugar-free candy/*Bonbon sans sucre*: candy only made of sweetener.

Sugar-free chewing gum★★★/*Chewing-gum sans sucre*: sweetened substance designed to be chewed.

Sugar-free chocolate spread/*Pâte chocolatée à tartiner sans sucre*: sugar-free, but sweetened, and very fat mix of chocolate and crushed hazelnuts.

Sugar-free cookie/*Biscuit sans sucre*: sweetened cookie. Carbohydrate.

Sugar-free ketchup/*Ketchup sans sucre*: thick spicy sauce made of tomatoes and sweetener.

Sugar-free plain muesli/*Muesli nature sans sucre*: mix of cereal flakes without added sugar. Carbohydrate.

Sugar-free skimmed powder cow's milk★★★/*Lait de vache écrémé en poudre sans sucre*: dehydrated skimmed cow's milk without added sugar.

Sugar-free skimmed powder goat milk★★★/*Lait de chèvre écrémé en poudre sans sucre*: dehydrated skimmed goat milk without added sugar.

Sugar-free skimmed powder sheep milk★★★/*Lait de brebis écrémé en poudre sans sucre*: dehydrated skimmed sheep milk without added sugar.

Sugar-free soda★★★/*Soda zéro*: fizzy beverage made of water, gas and one or several sweetener(s).

Sugar-free whole cow's milk in powder★★★/*Lait de vache entier en poudre sans sucre*: dehydrated whole cow's milk without added sugar.

Sugar-free whole goat milk in powder★★★/*Lait de chèvre entier en poudre sans sucre*: dehydrated whole goat milk without added sugar.

Sugar-free whole sheep milk in powder★★★/*Lait de brebis entier en poudre sans sucre*: dehydrated whole sheep milk without added sugar.

Sumac★★★/*Sumac*: spice with a salty aftertaste.

Sunchoke★★★/*Topinambour*: vegetable plant from which we eat the tubers. Green vegetable.
Note: do not eat canned vegetables (unless low in salt).

Sunchoke chips/*Chips de topinambour*: very thinly cut sunchoke, fried and salted.

Sunflower oil★★★/*Huile de tournesol*: fatty substance made of sunflower seeds.

Sunflower seed★★★/*Graine de tournesol*: sunflower seed eaten grilled.

Sunflower seed milk★★/*Lait de graines de tournesol*: plant milk from sunflower seeds. Lactose-free. *Note: do not consume it sweetened.*

Surimi/*Surimi*: mix of fish flesh flavored with crab.

Sushi/*Sushi*: small rice ball wrapped with raw fish cut in thin slices and wrapped in a seaweed leaf.

Sushi sauce/*Sauce sushi*: fermented soy sauce.

Swaledale cheese: raw cow's milk cheese. Dairy product.

Sweat/*Etuvée (à l')*: cf. "Steam".

Sweet and sour sauce/*Sauce aigre douce*: tomato sauce lightly sweetened.

Sweet chestnut cream/*Crème de marron*: sweet chestnut spread.

Sweet corn kernel/Maïs doux en grain: cereal from which we eat the cooked kernel. Carbohydrate. Gluten-free.

Sweet potato★★★/*Patate douce*: edible tuber. Carbohydrate.

Sweet potatoes chips/*Chips de patates douces*: very thinly cut sweet potatoes, fried and salted.

Sweet potato flour★★★/*Farine de patate douce*: powder made of the extraction of starch from sweet potatoes. Carbohydrate. Gluten-free.

Sweet shortcrust pastry/*Pâte sablée*: pastry made of flour, sugar, butter and eggs.

Sweet wine
- Sweetened skimmed powder cow's milk

Sweet wine/*Vin moelleux*: white wine which contains between 10 and 45 grams of sugar per liter.

Sweetened and semi-skimmed powder cow's milk/*Lait de vache demi-écrémé en poudre sucré*: dehydrated semi-skimmed cow's milk with added sugar.

Sweetened and semi-skimmed powder goat milk/*Lait de chèvre demi-écrémé en poudre sucré*: dehydrated semi-skimmed goat milk with added sugar.

Sweetened and semi-skimmed powder sheep milk/*Lait de brebis demi-écrémé en poudre sucré*: dehydrated semi-skimmed sheep milk with added sugar.

Sweetened condensed milk/*Lait concentré sucré*: agri-food transformation of the milk from the industry packed in metal box or in tube and sweetened.

Sweetened shoyu/*Shoyu sucré*: fermented and sweetened soy bean sauce.

Sweetened skimmed cow's milk yogurt/*Yaourt au lait de vache maigre sucré*: cow's milk which has been partially or completely skimmed before being fermented thanks to lactic acid bacteria and sweetened. Dairy product.

Sweetened skimmed goat milk yogurt/*Yaourt au lait de chèvre maigre sucré*: goat milk which has been partially or completely skimmed before being fermented thanks to lactic acid bacteria and sweetened. Dairy product.

Sweetened skimmed powder goat milk/*Lait de chèvre écrémé en poudre sucré*: dehydrated skimmed goat milk with added sugar.

Sweetened skimmed powder cow's milk/*Lait de vache écrémé en poudre sucré*: dehydrated skimmed cow's milk with added sugar.

Sweetened skimmed powder sheep milk/*Lait de brebis écrémé en poudre sucré*: dehydrated skimmed sheep milk with added sugar.

Sweetened skimmed sheep milk yogurt/*Yaourt au lait de brebis maigre sucré*: sheep milk which has been partially or completely skimmed before being fermented thanks to lactic acid bacteria and sweetened. Dairy product.

Sweetened whole cow's milk in powder/*Lait de vache entier en poudre sucré*: dehydrated whole cow's milk with added sugar.

Sweetened whole goat milk in powder/*Lait de chèvre entier en poudre sucré*: dehydrated whole goat milk with added sugar.

Sweetened whole goat milk yogurt/*Yaourt au lait de chèvre entier nature sucré*: whole goat milk fermented thanks to lactic acid bacteria before being sweetened. Dairy product.

Sweetened whole sheep milk in powder/*Lait de brebis entier en poudre sucré*: dehydrated whole sheep milk with added sugar.

Sweetened whole sheep milk yogurt/*Yaourt au lait de brebis entier nature sucré*: whole sheep milk fermented thanks to lactic acid bacteria before being sweetened. Dairy product.

Sweetened 0% fat fruit yogurt★★★/*Yaourt aux fruits à 0% de matière grasse édulcoré*: skimmed cow's milk, goat milk or sheep milk fermented thanks to lactic acid bacteria and in which fruits have been added. Dairy product.

Sweetened 0% fat yogurt★★★/*Yaourt à 0% de matière grasse édulcoré*: skimmed cow's milk, goat milk or sheep milk fermented thanks to lactic acid bacteria before being sweetened, usually with fructose. Dairy product.

Sweetener★★★/*Edulcorant*: substance suggesting the taste of sugar without containing sugar. Acaloric.

Swiss cheese: pasteurised cow's milk cheese. Dairy product.

Swiss dried beef/*Viande des grisons*: dried meat served in very thin slice.

Swordfish★★★/*Espadon*: fatty fish we can find in hot waters.

Syrup/*Sirop*: solution made of water and sugar.

T

Tabasco/Tabasco: chili pepper purée.

Tabbouleh★★/*Taboulé*: mix of wheat semolina, tomatoes, onions, bell peppers, raisins and mint leaves with olive oil. Carbohydrate.
Note: many commercially prepared foods are high in salt: prepare it yourself without salt and with authorized foods.

Table salt/*Sel de table*: sodium chloride used to season dishes.

Taco/*Taco*: corn flour crepe stuffed with meat, cheese and hot sauce. Carbohydrate. Gluten-free.

Tagine★/*Tagine*: dish made of pieces of meat or fish braised with green vegetables and various dried fruits.
Note: many commercially prepared foods are high in salt: prepare it yourself without salt and with authorized foods.

Tahini/*Tahini*: cf. "Sesame cream".

Tamari/*Tamari*: cf. "Soy sauce".

Tamarillo★★★/*Tamarillo*: small exotic fruit from the tamarillo.

Tamarind fruit in light syrup★/*Tamarin au sirop léger*: poached tamarind fruit preserved in more or less sugary water. Exotic fruit.

Tamarind fruit in syrup/*Tamarin au sirop*: poached tamarind fruit preserved in very sugary water. Exotic fruit.

Tanacetum balsamita★★★/*Balsamite*: plant which leaves you can use as a condiment.

Tango/*Tango*: beverage made of half beer and half grenadine syrup.

Tapenade/*Tapenade*: condiment made of crushed black olives, capers and anchovies with olive oil.

Tapioca★★★/*Tapioca*: cassava starch. Gluten-free.

Tapioca pearl★★★/*Perle du japon*: pearl made of cassava starch.

Tap water★★★/*Eau du robinet*: water commonly drunk and coming from the faucet.

Taramasalata/*Tarama*: mix of salted fish eggs, olive oil, bread crumb and lemon juice.

Taro(1)★★★/*Colocase*: tropical plant which edible rhizome is rich in starch and assimilated to a carbohydrate.

Taro(2)★★★/**Taro**: tropical plant grown for its edible tuber. Green vegetable.

Tarragon★★★/**Estragon**: aromatic plant used as a condiment.

Tartare of fatty fish★★★/**Poisson gras tartare**: ground fatty fish eaten raw.
Note: do not salt. A few fish are ★★.

Tartare of lean fish★★★/**Poisson maigre tartare**: ground lean fish eaten raw.
Note: do not salt. A few fish are ★★.

Tartar sauce/Sauce tartare: very seasoned mayonnaise with onions, capers and herbs.

Tartiflette/Tartiflette: dish made of melted reblochon, potatoes, lardons and onions.

Teal★★★/**Sarcelle**: wild duck. Game.

Teff flake★★★/**Flocon de teff**: small portion of dehydrated teff. Carbohydrate.

Teff flour★★★/**Farine de teff**: powder made of not whole-grain teff seed milling. Gluten-free.

Teleme cheese: pasteurised cow's milk cheese. Dairy product.

Tempeh/Tempeh: food product made of fermented mung beans.

Tench★★★/**Tanche**: freshwater fish with white flesh.

Tête-de-Maure cheese/Tête-de-Maure: cow's milk cheese wrapped in red paraffin wax. Dairy product.

Theine-free (tea)★★★/*Déthéiné (thé)*: tea from which the theine has been removed.
Note: do not drink it sweetened.

Thyme★★★/*Thym*: plant used as a spice.

Tilsit cheese/*Tilsit*: hard cow's milk cheese. Dairy product.

Tinned shoulder★★★/*Noix d'épaule*: canned pork shoulder.

Tiramisu/*Tiramisu*: dessert made of alternating layers of whipped mascarpone with egg yolks and cookies soaked in coffee, sprinkled with cocoa in powder.

Toast(1)/*Pain grillé*: fresh white bread cut in slices and industrially or "homemade" toasted. Carbohydrate.

Toast(2)/*Toast*: slice of toasted bread.

Toasted brioche/*Toast brioché*: slice of toasted brioche.

To fry★★★/*Frire*: to cook food in a boiling fatty substance.

Tofu/*Tofu*: poached or grilled soybean dough.

Tofu sausage/*Saucisse de tofu*: sausage made of soybean and vegetable oil.

Tomato★★★/*Tomate*: vegetable plant producing this fruit considered as a green vegetable: tomato. Green vegetable.

Tomato juice/*Jus de tomate*: juice made of the pressing of tomatoes.

Tomato paste★★★/*Concentré de tomate*: tomato purée sold in cans or in cartons.

Tomme de Brach/*Tomme de Brach*: cow's milk cheese with parsley in it. Dairy product.

Tomme de Romans/*Tomme de Romans*: soft cow's milk cheese. Dairy product.

Tomme de Savoie/*Tomme de Savoie*: pressed raw cow's milk cheese. Dairy product.

Topside★★/*Tende de tranche*: piece of beef to simmer. Red meat.

Tortilla★★/*Tortilla*: small crepe made of corn flour. Carbohydrate. Gluten-free.
Note: many commercially prepared foods are high in salt and/or in sugar so prepare it yourself without salt and sugar and with authorized foods.

Tortilla chips/*Tortilla chips*: swollen and light biscuit for the aperitif.

Tripe/*Tripes*: dish made of the stomach and various animal entrails as well as animal feet prepared in various ways. Offal.

Triple cream cheese★/*Fromage triple crème*: cheese containing more than 75% of fats. Dairy product.
Note: almost all cheeses are too salty.

Tripoux/*Tripoux*: dish made of mutton tripe simmered in sauce. Offal.

Trotter★★★/*Pied de porc*: pork foot. Offal.

Trout★★/*Truite*: fatty freshwater fish.

Trout eggs/*Œufs de truite*: trout eggs preserved in brine.

True cardamom★★★/*Cardamone*: spice.

True fera★★★/*Féra*: freshwater fish with white flesh.

Truffle★★★/*Truffe*: edible underground mushroom. Green vegetable.

Tuberose parsley★★★/*Persil à grosse racine*: vegetable plant grown for its edible root. Green vegetable.

Tuberous-roated chervil: cf. "Chaerophyllum b."

**Tuna and mayonnaise/*Thon à la mayonnaise*: tuna in a can with mayonnaise sauce.

**Tuna in Catalan sauce/*Thon à la catalane*: tuna in a can with Catalan sauce.

Tuna in oil★★★/*Thon à l'huile*: tuna in a can with vegetable oil.

**Tuna in tomato sauce/*Thon à la tomate*: tuna in a can with concentrated tomato sauce.

**Tuna rillettes/*Rillettes de thon*: cooked meat made of tuna cooked in vegetable oil.

Turkey★★★/*Dinde*: poultry with white flesh.

**Turkey and cheese escalope/*Cordon bleu de dinde*: turkey escalope wrapped around ham and cheese.

**Turkey chick (roast)/*Dindonneau (rôti de)*: roast made of lean turkey slices. Poultry.

Turkey tournedos★★★/*Tournedos de dinde*: round slice of turkey poult roast.

**Turkish delight/*Loukoum*: very sugary Eastern confection made of a pasted flavored with almonds, pistachios, etc.

Turmeric★★★/*Curcuma*: spice.

Turnip★★★/*Navet*: vegetable plant from which we eat the edible root. Green vegetable.

Turnip seed★★★/*Graine de navet*: turnip seed eaten crushed or germinated.

$\mathcal{U}$

UHT sterilized milk★★★/*Lait stérilisé UHT*: milk which has been thermally treated at 240°F during 15 seconds before being rapidly cooled.

Ullucus★★★/*Ulluque*: edible tuber of the olluco. Green vegetable.

Umbrina★★★/*Ombrine*: saltwater fish with white flesh.

Unleavened bread/*Pain azyme*: bread without leaven nor yeast. Carbohydrate.

Unsalted butter★★★/*Beurre doux*: unsalted dietary fats made from the cream of cow's milk.

$\mathcal{V}$

Vacherin(1)/*Vacherin(1)*: soft cow's milk cheese with washed rind. Dairy product.

Vacherin(2)/*Vacherin(2)*: half hard cow's milk cheese. Dairy product.

Valençay cheese/*Valençay*: raw goat milk cheese in the shape of a pyramid. Dairy product.

Vanilla★★★/*Vanille*: fruit from the vanilla planifolia used to flavor pastries.

Vanilla sugar/*Sucre vanillé*: sugar with vanilla extracts.

Varech/*Kelp*: edible seaweed.

Veal and cheese escalope/*Cordon bleu de veau*: veal escalope wrapped around ham and cheese.

Veal breast★★★/*Poitrine de veau*: inferior part of the veal's rib cage to boil or to simmer.

Veal fillet★★★/*Quasi de veau*: piece from the veal leg.

Veal gristle★★★/*Tendron de veau*: part of the veal composed of the cartilages which prolong the ribs.

Veal kidney★★/*Rognon de veau*: kidney of the veal. Offal.

Veal knuckle★★★/*Jarret de veau*: part of the leg behind the veal's knee joint. Meat to boil.

Veal liver★★★/*Foie de veau*: offal.

Veal loin★★★/*Longe de veau*: veal meat corresponding to the upper part of the cervical and lumbar areas.

Veal (meat)/*Veau (viande de...)*: all unprepared nor transformed meats, plain, ready to be cooked and cut from veal. See each piece separately.

Veal neck★★★/*Collet de veau*: piece of veal meat to boil.

Veal quenelle/*Quenelle de veau*: veal stuffing thickened with eggs and bread crumb before being shaped in sausage.

Veal rib★★★/Côte de veau: piece of veal meat to grill.

Veal rump★★★/*Culotte de veau*: piece of veal to roast.

Veal scallop★★★/*Noix de veau*: piece of veal served roasted or as a scallop.

Veal spare ribs★★★/*Carré de veau*: piece of veal meat to simmer.

Veal stock★★/*Fond de veau*: brown stock made of veal stock.
Note: many commercially prepared foods are high in salt: prepare it yourself without salt and with authorized foods.

Veal sweetbread★★★/*Ris de veau*: veal thymus. Offal.

Vegan★★/*Végétalien(ne)*: person who does not eat any animal-based food.
Note: many commercially prepared foods are high in salt: prepare it yourself without salt and with authorized foods.

Vegetable fondue★★/*Fondue de légumes*: dish made of vegetables slowly cooked in a fatty substance.
Note: many commercially prepared foods are high in salt: prepare it yourself without salt and with authorized foods.

Vegetable fry fat★★★/*Graisse à frire végétale*: block of vegetable fat, especially coconut oil and palm kernel oil, used to fry food.

Vegetable gelatin/*Gélatine végétale*: cf. "Agar-agar".

Vegetable julienne★★★/*Julienne de légumes*: mix of green vegetable cut in thin sticks.
Note: do not eat canned vegetables (unless low in salt).

Vegetable pancake to pan-fry/*Galette végétale à poêler*: food under the form of a steak made of cereals: quinoa and/or wheat and/or rice, etc. without meat.

Vegetable steak/*Steak végétal*: cereal steak made of wheat and/or quinoa and/or soybean, etc. Meatless.

Vegetable terrine★★/*Pain de légumes*: dish made of potatoes, green vegetables, butter and eggs served cold with a mayonnaise.
Note: many commercially prepared foods are high in salt: prepare it yourself without salt and with authorized foods.

Vegetarian oyster sauce/*Sauce d'huître végétarienne*: sauce made of shiitakes (black mushrooms) stock reduction.

Vegetarian★★/*Végétarien(ne)*: person who does not eat meat nor fish nor any transformed dish or product containing meat or fish.
Note: many commercially prepared foods are high in salt: prepare it yourself without salt and with authorized foods.

Venison (meat)★★/*Chevreuil (viande de...)*: red meat and game.

Venison★★/*Venaison*: edible flesh from big games (wild boar, deer, hind, etc.)

Ventreche★★★/*Ventrèche*: lean lard.

Verbena★★★/*Verveine*: plant used as a condiment and eaten in infusions.
Note: do not drink it sweetened.

Vermicelli(1)/*Vermicelle*: sweetened chestnut pasta in the shape of a thin filament.

Vermicelli(2)/*Vermicelle de "..."*: cf. ""..." pasta".

Very rare/*Bleu*: cooking method during which the red meat remains bloody.

Vienna bread/*Pain viennois*: bread which batter contains sugar, milk, fats and eggs.

193

Viennoiserie/*Viennoiserie*: bakery product made of a fermented dough with milk, sugar, fats and eggs.

Vieux-Lille cheese/*Vieux-Lille*: very fermented raw cow's milk cheese. Dairy product.

Vila-vila★★★/*Morelle de Balbis*: plant from which we eat the small fruits.

Vinaigrette sauce★★★/*Sauce vinaigrette*: sauce made of vegetable oil and vinegar.

Vinegar★★★/*Vinaigre*: aqueous sour solution made of a fermented alcoholic beverage.

Vodka/*Vodka*: eau de vie made of wheat and rye seeds.

W

Waffle★★/*Gaufre*: light honeycombed pastry.
Note: many commercially prepared foods are high in salt and/or in sugar so prepare it yourself without salt and sugar and with authorized foods.

Wakame/*Wakamé*: edible seaweed.

Wakame pasta/*Pâte alimentaire de wakamé*: mix to be cooked made of wakame (edible seaweed). Green vegetable.

Walleye★★★/*Doré*: freshwater fish very similar to zander.

Walnut★★★/*Noix*: nut from the walnut tree.

Walnut oil★★★/*Huile de noix*: fatty substance made of walnut.

Warp/*Warp*: sieved wheat pancake. Carbohydrate.

Wasabi/*Wasabi*: Japanese mustard.

Watercress★★★/*Cresson*: plant grown for its edible leaves. Green vegetable.

Watercress seed★★★/*Graine de cresson*: watercress seed eaten crushed or germinated.

Waterloo cheese: raw cow's milk cheese. Dairy product.

Watermelon in light syrup★/*Pastèque au sirop léger*: poached watermelon preserved in more or less sugary water.

Watermelon in syrup/*Pastèque au sirop*: poached watermelon preserved in very sugary water.

Watermelon juice★★/*Jus de pastèque*: juice made of the pressing of watermelons.

Wax bean★★/*Haricot beurre*: yellow bean eaten young. Green vegetable.

Wedge sole★/*Céteau*: small sole, flat saltwater fish with white flesh.

Weever★★★/*Vive*: saltwater fish with white flesh.

Wheat bran★★★/*Son de blé*: residue of wheat milling.

Wheat bread industrially toasted/*Pain de froment grillé industriel*: white bread slice industrially toasted.

Wheat crispbread/*Biscotte de froment*: slice of sandwich bread industrially toasted in the oven. Carbohydrate.

Wheat germ oil★★★/*Huile de germe de blé*: fatty substance made of wheat germ.

Wheat gluten/*Seitan*: food product made of wheat proteins.

Wheat pasta★★★/*Pâte alimentaire de blé*: mix to be cooked made of refined hard wheat semolina. Carbohydrate.

Wheat tunnbröd/*Pain suédois au froment*: small dry bread made of soft wheat flour. Carbohydrate.

Wheat(1)★★★/*Blé(1)*: herbaceous plant from which the grain is extracted to make wheat flour used to make bread and pasta, etc. Carbohydrate.

Wheat(2)★★★/*Blé(2)*: pre-cooked whole wheat. Carbohydrate.

Wheat★★★/*Froment*: soft wheat. Carbohydrate.

Wheatgerm★★★/*Germe de blé*: wheat germ sold loose.

Whelk/*Bulot* : sea shellfish.

Whipped cream/*Crème Chantilly*: whipped crème fraîche with sugar.

Whipped egg whites★★/*Œuf monté en neige*: egg white whipped until firm and foamy.
Note: many commercially prepared foods are high in salt: prepare it yourself without salt.

Whipping cream★★★/*Crème fleurette*: cream with 10 to 12% of fats. Made of sterilized UHT milk. Dairy product.

Whiskey/*Whisky*: grain eau de vie.

White barley flour★★★/*Farine d'orge blanche*: powder made of not whole-grain barley milling. Carbohydrate.

White bread/*Pain blanc*: bread made of white or sieved flour. Carbohydrate.

White bread crumb/*Mie de pain blanc*: bread made of white flour without its crust. Carbohydrate.

White buckwheat flour★★★/*Farine de sarrasin blanche*: powder made of not whole-grain buckwheat milling. Carbohydrate.

White chocolate/*Chocolat blanc*: confection made of fats, dairy products and sugar. Does not contain cocoa powder.

White einkorn wheat flour★★★/*Farine de petit épeautre blanche*: powder made of not whole-grain einkorn wheat milling. Carbohydrate.

White flour★★★/*Farine blanche*: flour made of grains without their peel. Only starch is kept. It is thus very poor in fiber. T45 to T80 flour in Europe. Carbohydrate.

White fonio★★★/*Fonio*: very thin grain. Carbohydrate. Gluten-free.

White fonio flake★★★/*Flocon de fonio*: small portion of dehydrated white fonio. Carbohydrate. Gluten-free.

White meat★★★/*Viande blanche*: poultry, veal, pork, rabbit meat.

White millet flour★★★/*Farine de millet blanche*: powder made of not whole-grain millet milling. Carbohydrate.

White oats flour★★★/*Farine d'avoine blanche*: powder made of not wholewheat oats milling. Carbohydrate.

White rice★★★/*Riz blanc*: rice without peel and without bran. Carbohydrate. Gluten-free.

White rye flour★★★/*Farine de seigle blanche*: powder made of not whole-grain rye milling. Carbohydrate.

White sauce★★/*Sauce blanche*: white roux made of butter and flour.
Note: many commercially prepared foods are high in salt: prepare it yourself without salt.

White sausage/*Boudin blanc*: cooked meat made of lean meat stuffing, milk, eggs, cream, bread crumbs or flour and spices.

White spelt flour★★★/*Farine d'épeautre blanche*: powder made of not whole-grain spelt milling. Carbohydrate.

White sugar/*Sucre blanc*: very sugary substance extracted from sugar cane and/or sugar beet. Fast-acting sugar.

White tea★★★/*Thé blanc*: infusion of white tea leaves.
Note: do not drink it sweetened.

White wheat flour★★★/*Farine de blé blanche*: powder made of not wholewheat milling. Carbohydrate.

White wine★/*Vin blanc*: wine made thanks of the grape must alcoholic fermentation.
Note: do not drink alcoholic beverage, however no problem if it's cooked.

Whiting★★★/*Merlan*: saltwater fish with white flesh.

Whole cow's milk★★★/*Lait de vache entier*: cow's milk which has not been skimmed.

Whole goat milk★★★/*Lait de chèvre entier*: goat milk which has not been skimmed.

Whole sheep milk★★★/*Lait de brebis entier*: sheep milk which has not been skimmed.

Whole tomato preserved peeled/*Tomate entière pelée en conserve*: peeled tomato preserved in brine.

Whole-grain almond purée★★★/*Purée d'amande complète*: mashed whole-grain almonds to spread.

Whole-grain and gluten-free bagel/*Bagel complet sans gluten*: small whole-grain bread shaped into a ring with very firm gluten-free crumb. Carbohydrate.

Whole-grain bagel/*Bagel complet*: small whole-grain bread shaped into a ring with very firm crumb. Carbohydrate.

Whole-grain barley flake★★★/*Flocon d'orge complète*: small portion of dehydrated whole-grain barley. Carbohydrate.

Whole-grain barley flour★★★/*Farine d'orge complète*: powder made of whole-grain barley milling. Carbohydrate.

Whole-grain breakfast cookie/*Biscuit pour petit-déjeuner riche en céréales complètes*: cookie rich in whole grains and adapted to breakfast. Carbohydrate.

Whole-grain buckwheat cornflakes/*Corn flakes de sarrasin complet*: grilled flakes made of whole-grain buckwheat flakes. Carbohydrate. Gluten-free.

Whole-grain buckwheat flake★★★/*Flocon de sarrasin complet*: small portion of dehydrated whole-grain buckwheat. Carbohydrate.

Whole-grain buckwheat flour★★★/*Farine de sarrasin complète*: powder made of whole-grain buckwheat milling. Carbohydrate.

**Whole-grain buckwheat pancake
- Whole-grain fajita**

Whole-grain buckwheat pancake/*Galette complète*: flat, thin and round dish made of whole-grain buckwheat flour, eggs and milk cooked in a frying pan. Carbohydrate. Gluten-free.

Whole-grain cannellonis/*Cannelloni complet*: whole-grain pasta rolled in the shape of a cylinder and stuffed with stuffing. Carbohydrate.

Whole-grain cashew purée★★★/*Purée de noix de cajou complète*: mashed whole-grain cashew to spread.

Whole-grain corn cornflakes/*Corn flakes de maïs complet*: grilled flakes made of whole-grain corn corn flakes. Carbohydrate. Gluten-free.

Whole-grain corn flake★★★/*Flocon de maïs complet*: small portion of dehydrated whole-grain corn. Carbohydrate. Gluten-free.

Whole-grain corn flour★★★/*Farine de maïs complète*: powder made of whole-grain corn milling. Carbohydrate. Gluten-free.

Whole-grain crispbread/*Biscotte complète*: slice of whole-grain sandwich bread industrially toasted in the oven. Carbohydrate.

Whole-grain einkorn wheat flake★★★/*Flocon de petit-épeautre complet*: small portion of dehydrated whole-grain einkorn wheat. Carbohydrate.

Whole-grain einkorn wheat flour★★★/*Farine de petit épeautre complet*: powder made of whole-grain einkorn wheat milling. Carbohydrate.

Whole-grain fajita/*Fajita complète*: whole-grain corn tortilla. Carbohydrate. Gluten-free.

Whole-grain fonio flake★★★/*Flocon de fonio complète*: small portion of dehydrated whole-grain fonio. Carbohydrate. Gluten-free.

Whole-grain frik★★★/*Frik complet*: crushed not fully grown whole-grain wheat. Carbohydrate.

Whole-grain gluten-free crispbread/*Biscotte complète sans gluten*: slice of whole-grain gluten-free sandwich bread industrially toasted in the oven. Carbohydrate.

Whole-grain gluten-free kringle/Craquelin complet sans *gluten*: small whole-grain crispy cookie made of an unleavened and gluten-free batter.

Whole-grain gnocchi/*Gnocchi complet:* ball made of wholewheat semolina and potatoes. Carbohydrate.

Whole-grain grissino/*Gressin complet*: small whole-grain bread made with an egg batter. Carbohydrate.

Whole-grain hazelnut purée★★★/*Purée de noisette complète*: mashed whole-grain hazelnuts to spread.

Whole-grain khorasan wheat flake★★★/*Flocon de kamut complet*: small portion of dehydrated whole-grain khorasan wheat. Carbohydrate.

Whole-grain khorasan wheat flour★★★/*Farine de kamut complète*: powder made of whole-grain khorasan wheat milling. Carbohydrate.

Whole-grain kringle/*Craquelin complet*: small whole-grain crispy cookie made of an unleavened batter.

Whole-grain millet flake★★★/*Flocon de millet complet*: small portion of dehydrated whole-grain millet. Carbohydrate. Gluten-free.

Whole-grain millet flour
- Whole-grain polenta

Whole-grain millet flour★★★/*Farine de millet complète*: powder made of whole-grain millet milling. Carbohydrate.

Whole-grain millet slice of bread/*Tartine craquante millet complète*: flat and light slice of bread made of whole-grain millet flour. Carbohydrate. Gluten-free.

Whole-grain milliasse★★/*Milliasse complète*: mash made of whole-grain corn flour before being cooled and grilled. Carbohydrate. Gluten-free.
Note: many commercially prepared foods are high in salt: prepare it yourself without salt and with authorized foods.

Whole-grain muffin/*Muffin complet*: small plain whole-grain bread with leaven. Carbohydrate.

Wholegrain mustard/*Moutarde à l'ancienne*: mustard with its seeds.

Whole-grain oats flour★★★/*Farine d'avoine complète*: powder made of whole-grain oats milling. Carbohydrate.

Whole-grain fonio flour★★★/*Farine de fonio complète*: powder made of whole-grain folio milling. Carbohydrate. Gluten-free.

Whole-grain peanut purée★★★/*Purée d'arachide complète*: mashed whole-grain peanuts to spread.

Whole-grain pistachio purée★★★/*Purée de pistache complète*: mashed whole-grain pistachios to spread.

Whole-grain polenta★★/*Polenta complète*: whole-grain corn mush. Gluten-free.
Note: many commercially prepared foods are high in salt: prepare it yourself without salt.

Whole-grain quinoa flour★★★/*Farine de quinoa complète*: flour made of whole-grain quinoa seed milling. Gluten-free.

Whole-grain rice★★★/*Riz complet*: rice eaten intact without its peel. Carbohydrate. Gluten-free.

Whole-grain rice bulgur★★★/*Boulgour de riz complet*: crushed whole-grain rice steamed or cooked in water. Carbohydrate. Gluten-free.

Whole-grain rice cornflakes/*Corn flakes de riz complet*: grilled flakes made of whole-grain rice flakes. Carbohydrate. Gluten-free.

Whole-grain rice cream★★★/*Crème de riz complet*: more or less liquid cream made of whole-grain rice milk, substitute to crème fraîche.

Whole-grain rice flake★★★/*Flocon de riz complet*: small portion of dehydrated whole-grain rice. Carbohydrate. Gluten-free.

Whole-grain rice flour★★★/*Farine de riz complet*: powder made of whole-grain rice milling. Carbohydrate. Gluten-free.

Whole-grain rye flake★★★/*Flocon de seigle complet*: small portion of dehydrated whole-grain rye. Carbohydrate.

Whole-grain rye flour★★★/*Farine de seigle complète*: powder made of whole-grain rye milling. Carbohydrate.

Whole-grain salt-free & gluten-free crispbread ★★★/*Biscotte complète sans sel & sans gluten*: slice of whole-grain gluten-free and salt-free sandwich bread industrially toasted in the oven. Carbohydrate.

Whole-grain soybean flake
- Wholewheat bread

Whole-grain soybean flake★★★/*Flocon de soja complet*: small portion of dehydrated whole-grain soybean. Carbohydrate.

Whole-grain soybean flour★★★/*Farine de soja complète*: flour made of whole-grain soybean milling. Gluten-free.

Whole-grain spelt cornflakes/*Corn flakes d'épeautre complet*: grilled flakes made of whole-grain spelt flakes. Carbohydrate.

Whole-grain spelt flake★★★/*Flocon d'épeautre complet*: small portion of dehydrated whole-grain spelt. Carbohydrate.

Whole-grain spelt flour★★★/*Farine d'épeautre complète*: powder from whole-grain spelt milling. Carbohydrate.

Whole-grain teff flake★★★/*Flocon de teff complet*: small portion of dehydrated whole-grain teff. Carbohydrate.

Whole-grain teff flour★★★/*Farine de teff complète*: flour made of whole-grain teff seed milling. Gluten-free.

Whole-grain tortilla★★/*Tortilla complète*: small crepe made of whole wheat corn flour. Carbohydrate. Gluten-free.
Note: many commercially prepared foods are high in salt and/or in sugar so prepare it yourself without salt and sugar and with authorized foods.

Whole-grain amaranth flour★★★/*Farine d'amarante complète*: flour made of whole-grain amaranth milling. Gluten-free.

Wholewheat bread/*Pain complet*: bread made of wholewheat or semi wholewheat flour. Carbohydrate.

Wholewheat bread crumb/*Mie de pain complet*: bread made of wholewheat flour without its crust. Carbohydrate.

Wholewheat breadcrumbs/*Chapelure complète*: wholewheat bread toasted in the oven before being crushed into crumbs. Carbohydrate.

Wholewheat bread industrially toasted/*Pain complet grillé industriel*: wholewheat bread slice industrially toasted.

Wholewheat bulgur★★★/*Boulgour complet*: crushed whole wheat steamed or cooked in water. Carbohydrate.

Wholewheat bun/*Bun complet*: small round and puffy wholewheat bread. Carbohydrate.

Wholewheat crepe★★/*Crêpe complète*: thin layer of cooked batter made of eggs, milk and wholewheat flour. Carbohydrate.
Note: many commercially prepared foods are high in salt and/or in sugar so prepare it yourself without salt and sugar and with authorized foods.

Wholewheat crouton/*Croûton complet*: small piece of fried wholewheat bread. Carbohydrate.

Wholemeal flour★★★/*Farine complète:* flour made of whole-grains or almost whole grains. It is thus rich in fiber.

Wholewheat flour(1)★★★/*Farine complète:* flour made of whole-grains or almost whole grains. It is thus rich in fiber.

Wholewheat flour(2)★★★/*Farine de blé complète*: powder made of wholewheat milling. Carbohydrate.

Wholewheat gluten-free bun
- Wild boar (meat)

Wholewheat gluten-free bun/*Bun complet sans gluten*: small round and puffy gluten-free wholewheat bread. Carbohydrate.

Wholewheat lasagna★★★/***Lasagne complète*: pasta made of wholewheat flour in the shape of large flat patches. Carbohydrate.

Wholewheat macaroni★★★/***Macaroni complet*: wholewheat semolina pasta in the shape of a tube. Carbohydrate.

Wholewheat pancakes★★/***Pancakes complet*: small thick crepes made of wholewheat flour. Carbohydrate. *Note: many commercially prepared foods are high in salt and/or in sugar so prepare it yourself without salt and sugar and with authorized foods.*

Wholewheat peanut flour★★★/***Farine d'arachide complète*: flour made of wholewheat peanut milling. Gluten-free.

Wholewheat pitta/*Pita complet*: unleavened wholewheat bread. Carbohydrate.

Wholewheat toast(1)/*Pain grillé complet*: fresh wholewheat bread cut in slices and industrially or "homemade" toasted. Carbohydrate.

Wholewheat toast(2)/*Toast complet*: slice of wholewheat toasted bread.

Wholewheat tunnbröd/*Pain suédois complet*: small dry bread made of wholewheat flour. Carbohydrate.

Wholewheat wrap/*Warp complet*: wholewheat pancake. Carbohydrate.

Wild boar (meat)★★★/***Sanglier (viande de...)*: untransformed and unprepared plain meats, ready to be cooked and coming from the wild boar. Game.

Wild rabbit★★/*Lapin sauvage*: herbivore mammal. Game.

Wild rice/*Riz sauvage*: cf. "Whole-grain rice".

Williamine★★★/*Williamine*: pear eau de vie.

Wine beef fondue★★/*Fondue bourguignonne au vin*: dish made of small dices of beef dipped in boiling wine. Red meat.

Winkle/*Bigorneau*: edible mollusk.

Winter purslane: cf. "Claytonia perfoliata".

X

Xylitol★★★/*Xylitol*: alcohol-sugar used as a sweetener.

Y

Yacón★★★/*Poire de terre*: vegetable plant from which we eat the tubers. Carbohydrate. Gluten-free.

Yakitori sauce/*Sauce yakitori*: fermented and sweetened soy sauce.

Yam★★★/*Igname*: vegetable plant grown for its rhizome. Green vegetable.

Yam flake★★★/*Flocon d'igname*: small portion of dehydrated yam. Carbohydrate.

Yam flour★★★/*Farine d'igname*: powder made of yam milling. Carbohydrate. Gluten-free.

Yannoh - 0% fat goat milk cottage cheese

Yannoh★★★/*Yannoh*: beverage made of rye, curly endive, acorn and barley.
Note: do not drink it sweetened.

Yogurt rich in phytosterol★★/*Yaourt riche en phytostérols*: cow's milk, goat milk or sheep milk fermented thanks to lactic acid bacteria before being enriched with phytosterol. Dairy product.
Note: do not consume it sweetened.

Yogurt with cereals/*Yaourt aux céréales*: sweetened yogurt with various cereals in powder.

Yogurt with muesli : cf. "Yogurt with cereals".

York ham/*Jambon d'York*: pork ham cooked with its bone. Cooked meat.

Young rooster★★★/*Coquelet*: young hen or young chicken. Poultry.

Z

Zander★★★/*Sandre*: freshwater fish with white flesh.

0% fat cow's milk cottage cheese★★★/*Faisselle au lait de vache à 0% de matière grasse*: fresh cheese made of skimmed cow's milk. Dairy product.

0% fat cow's milk fromage blanc★★★/*Fromage blanc de vache à 0% de matière grasse*: fresh cheese made of skimmed cow's milk, a bit drained and not aged. Dairy product.

0% fat goat milk cottage cheese★★★/*Faisselle au lait de chèvre à 0% de matière grasse*: fresh cheese made of skimmed goat milk. Dairy product.

**0% fat goat milk fromage blanc★★★/*Fromage blanc de chèvre à 0% de matière grasse*: fresh cheese made of skimmed goat milk, a bit drained and not aged. Dairy product.

**0% fat sheep milk cottage cheese★★★/*Faisselle au lait de brebis à 0% de matière grasse*: fresh cheese made of skimmed sheep milk. Dairy product.

**0% fat sheep milk fromage blanc★★★/*Fromage blanc de brebis à 0% de matière grasse*: fresh cheese made of skimmed sheep milk, a bit drained and not aged. Dairy product.

**0% fat yogurt with sugar/*Yaourt à 0% de matière grasse sucré*: skimmed cow's milk, goat milk or sheep milk fermented thanks to lactic acid bacteria and in which sugar is added. Dairy product.

**0% sugar syrup★★★/*Sirop 0% de sucre*: syrup made of sweetener, usually stevia extracts.

**Zerumbet★★★/*Zérumbet*: aromatic rhizome close to ginger. Green vegetable.

**Zest★★★/*Zeste*: external peel of citrus fruits.

**Zucchini★★★/*Courgette*: kind of squash with round and long fruit. Green vegetable.

All books by Ménard Cédric

Culinary dictionary for osteoporosis.
Culinary dictionary forcolonic diverticula.
Culinary dictionary for constipation.
Culinary dictionary for a food without gluten.
Culinary dictionary for anemia.
Culinary dictionary forangina pectoris.
Culinary dictionary for calcium oxalate kidney stones.
Culinary dictionary for corticosteroid therapy.
Culinary dictionary for diarrhea.
Culinary dictionary for diet without lactose.
Culinary dictionary for gastritis.
Culinary dictionary for gastroesophageal reflux disease.
Culinary dictionary for gout.
Culinary dictionary for hypercholesterolemia.
Culinary dictionary for heart failure.
Culinary dictionary for hemochromatosis.
Culinary dictionary for hiatal hernia.
Culinary dictionary for hypothyroidism.
Culinary dictionary for indigestion (or dyspepsia).
Culinary dictionary for lose weight.
Culinary dictionary for low sodium diet.
Culinary dictionary for myocardial infarction.
Culinary dictionary for breastfeeding.
Culinary dictionary of nutritional valueof food.
Culinary dictionary for diabetes mellitus.
Culinary dictionary for healthy pregnant woman.
Culinary dictionary for ulcerative colitis.
Culinary dictionary for uric acid kidney stones.
Culinary dictionary for theCrohn's disease.
Culinary dictionary for pancreatitis.
Culinary dictionary for cystic fibrosis.
Recipes and menusfor ulcerative colitis.
Recipes and menus for the Crohn's disease.

www.ingramcontent.com/pod-product-compliance
Lightning Source LLC
Chambersburg PA
CBHW070329220526
45467CB00001B/92